for XABIE

with friend

and deep connect

regard

Rachd

Sores/hoeo
7/8/2016

Rached Daoud is a Lebanese-born physician
and writer, now based in London. He
studied medicine at the American University
of Beirut and at Cluj-Napoca University in
Romania. He is known internationally for
his success in treating patients for whom
conventional medicine has no solutions.

DOCTOR IMPOSSIBLE

RACHED DAOUD

Cadmea Publishing
London 2016

ISBN 978-0-9934816-1-1

First published in Great Britian in 2015 by Cadmea
This revised and illustrated edition published in 2016
Copyright © Rached Daoud 2016

A CIP catalogue record for this book
is available from the British Library.

Illustrations by Rached Daoud © Rached Daoud 2016

Book cover - "Portrait of Dr. Daoud", oil on canvas
by Incze Daniel

Acknowledgements

I would like to express my appreciation to everyone who helped me with their comments and support to produce this book, and for all those who contributed to its editing, proofreading and design.

Table of Contents

Introduction

This book is about healing, about patients who were healed of incurable illness. It tells the story of my childhood spirituality, how I practised medicine during the Lebanese War and became known as a healer. I describe how difficult it was to help my patients and how love, like an angel, guided me to heal.

I started to write *Doctor Impossible* when I was suffering from a tumour in my right ear, hoping that it would inspire others. While writing about my struggle to heal my patients I saw how frustrated I had been. Frustration may have built up in me over the years, becoming the negative emotion underlying my illness and possibly even provoking the growth of my tumour. It took me a long time battling with all my fears, worries and anxieties until at last I came up with the idea of writing the book. In describing my patients' case histories and how they were healed, I learned from their example how to heal myself.

My journey started on Christmas morning 2006. I woke up feeling dizzy, with severe tinnitus and loss of hearing in my right ear. I felt drained of energy and my whole body ached. I had been working very hard as a doctor in Lebanon for over twenty years, often travelling to other countries to treat patients for whom medicine had not yet found a solution. My health deteriorated, so I went to see a doctor. He examined me, looked at my test results and told me that I had a neuroma which needed immediate surgery, otherwise I might soon die.

I am a physician who never gives up and cannot bear to leave my patients until they are healed. When no-one else can help them, I have to struggle to discover new solutions to their problems. I believe strongly in my healing ability. I'd met many terminally ill patients for whom doctors could do nothing; everyone, sometimes including me, expected them to die, but somehow they recovered. So why not try to find some way to heal myself and recover my hearing?

I decided to monitor the progress of my tumour while looking for non-surgical ways to cure it. If my condition continued to deteriorate I could always reconsider my decision to refuse surgery.

My family and friends heard about my problem and became very worried. They begged me to change my mind about an operation and were starting to drive me crazy. I dislike people feeling sorry for me. I'd never been seriously ill and had never needed help, but now I did. Perhaps I hadn't given enough of myself and fell ill because of that. The time had come for me to give my all. Would God heal me if I gave up everything? At the time I thought so.

I decided to leave Lebanon. But where to go? The best place for me was Romania. I knew the country well, spoke its language, had many friends there and would enjoy staying with them. So one moonless night I locked up my home near Beirut overlooking the sea in Jounieh and disappeared without a trace. I arrived the next morning in Bucharest feeling like a broken-down old warhorse. Many friends were waiting for me at the airport and as soon as my feet touched Romanian soil I felt a new zest for life.

But my tinnitus became louder and louder until it was unbearable. I didn't sleep for nights and couldn't bear being left alone. Wanting to take my problem less seriously and not make such a drama out of it, I decided to spend time with my friends and have fun. My Romanian friends know how to have a good laugh. Perhaps humour was the solution to my problem. So we partied nightly until morning. Their laughter distracted me from the noises in my head; it was as if I had my own private orchestra and I started to enjoy myself again. How could I get them excited enough to make them want to be with me all the time?

The answer was to invite everyone to an non-stop open healing party with plenty of food and drink. Day and night, a crowd of us moved from place to place all over Romania. I gave endless speeches and used my hands to heal everyone, whether they were sick or not. In my euphoria, I started to wonder what was so wrong with being able to hear in only one ear. I could always turn the deaf ear to anyone I didn't want to listen to. With both ears I'd have to hear both good and bad news, but with only one good ear I would hear only the good news.

What was wrong with having tinnitus, anyway? The gushing noises were similar to the sound of a waterfall. I love the rush of running water. It always reminds me of the beautiful waterfall near my native village in the green valleys of Lebanon.

At the end of my Romanian adventure I felt wonderful. My symptoms were no longer bothering me, but the time had come to return to Lebanon for another medical check-up, to see how my neuroma was progressing. I left Romania happy and went for an MRI scan as soon as I arrived in Beirut. The results were encouraging: the tumour had stopped growing and was stable. In my medical opinion, I no longer needed an operation, since there was no risk of it growing and pressing on my brain. But wanting a second opinion, just in case, I took the test results to my doctor.

After looking at them and examining me for five minutes he smiled, shook his head and told me that my tumour was in temporary remission but could start to grow again at any time. As I left his clinic I slammed the door behind me. Anxious and starting to feel unwell again, I resolved to shut up my home for the last time and I left for England.

There was nothing for me to do in London except look after myself. Boredom drove me crazy, so I started to write a book. I wanted to see my reality and beyond so as to understand how to heal myself, and began to ask myself why I had always longed for everyone to be happy. Did I have to sacrifice myself like an idealist, always frustrating myself with my unrealistic altruism? Was it really worth making such a huge effort to pursue my far-off dream? Why couldn't I simply accept the reality of the world as it was and live a normal life like everyone else?

Perhaps my frustration had nothing to do with my medical principles or practice and was instead due to my traumatic childhood. I suffered much as a child and had to protect myself by escaping to the wilderness, where I could find inner peace and security. I felt very vulnerable and sought a better world filled with love, asking my angels to rescue my troubled soul.

When I grew up I hoped to create a world of true humanity and decided to study medicine. As I started to practise as a doctor I became more idealistic than ever and turned my practice into an art full of love, looking for refuge from worldliness through altruism, compassion and healing.

Then why was I so frustrated? What's wrong with wanting to change the world through healing others? I can't bear to see their suffering; it reminds me of my own frustration, rooted in my childhood. Was I hanging on to it so I could apply it to my patients' frustration to heal all our frustration? Had I been trying to apply my pain to their pain to heal all pain?

Whenever I meet a sick person, I feel I must make them happy by freeing them quickly from their misery before it reflects itself onto me, triggering my own. I always believed that serving my patients by relieving their pain would support my idealism so that I could heal my own trauma while healing the world. Had my patients kidnapped my soul, using up all my time and energy as I attempted to heal them and make them happy? Is that what caused my endless frustration?

Surely not. How could I possibly believe that my poor patients were preventing me from living a normal life? It was my own choice to become a doctor and to devote myself to healing others.

Was it all my parents' fault? They had always wanted me to raise a family and be successful and earn lots of money. My mother saw how I neglected myself, sacrificing my life for the sake of others, and was sad that I wasn't looking after myself and had no wife and children. She tried to make me understand, but had to accept how stubborn I was and finally stopped worrying about me. She blessed me before her death, saying that God would look after me for the many good things I had given others.

My father hated to see my lack of interest in wealth and luxury. He warned me not to be an idealistic fool and to get rich instead. When he saw how rigid I was and unable to change my mind, he admonished me and told me a traditional parable.

Once upon a time, a doctor was wandering through the forest when he heard a moan coming from the other side of a steep hill. He thought it might be someone in trouble who needed his help and looked around to see who it was. It was the Devil, who had fallen from the top of the hill and was badly injured. He begged the doctor to carry him to hospital.

The doctor ignored the Devil and started to walk away, since curing him was completely against his principles. The Devil smiled and asked him how he could make a living without a devil to create illness and suffering. The doctor admitted his need to keep the Devil alive and immediately carried him to hospital.

I asked my father, "Are you telling me that I should carry the Devil and care for him because I need him to make healthy people sick so I can make money out of them?"

"Of course I am!" he replied. "You have to live. The people coming to you today are here only because they need you. They applaud your generosity and flatter you simply to benefit from you materially, steal your energy and manipulate you emotionally. One day when you are old, weak, tired, poor, drained and no longer able to give, how will you be able to go on living? You'll end up like a wretched dog. You are not saving money for your dark days and have no family to look after you. If you then ask for help from those who say they love you, I'm certain that no one will bother even to pee on your wounded finger! They will have no more use for you and you'll be nothing but a big headache for them."

"Well," I declared, "I refuse to carry the Devil."

"Then, my dear son, the Devil will have to carry you!"

From childhood my life has been devoted to serving humanity and I'm not about to change now. What use is life without principles? I am what I am. I'm neither victim nor hero; I am just here for others, simply a human being.

As I continued to write my stories, I saw how vain I had been and how arrogantly I had often behaved. I was unable to heal myself with my scientific scepticism, always looking for rational explanations for everything.

Writing about my patients, I saw how their humility helped them to be cured. Those of them who had recovered from terminal illness were full of childlike faith and trust. They were full, too, of inner peace and acceptance, free of doubt, grateful to live in a positive, creative simplicity and able quickly and easily to enter a blissful state. I was the opposite. Dogmatic, authoritarian, over-idealistic and judgemental, I couldn't get out of my head and simply be.

My patients who are healed are full of hope. They leave behind their past frustrations and surrender peacefully to the healing present. They fall in love with themselves, without expectation or neediness. All their fears dissipate and they accept life as it comes. They see beauty in everything and understand the real message behind illness. They are able to turn their negative emotions into positive ones, their fearfulness into a courageous love of life, anxiety into inner peace, and depression into humility. Their defensiveness turns into self-esteem and confidence; complaint into gratitude; apathy into selflessness; emotional and mental rigidity into tolerance, adaptability and flexibility; confusion and delusion into clarity and vigilance; insecurity into serenity; victimisation into resilience and reconciliation; self-absorption into insight and generosity; self-abuse and martyrdom into bravery and freedom; addiction into independence and ruthlessness into compassion.

My book is written and now I see it all. My black clouds have lifted, the darkness in my soul has gone. A new dawn is rising within me. I am renewed and filled with light. The beauty of healing is descending upon me. The anonymous doctor has come from beyond to cure my impossibility. It is he who is Doctor Impossible. Everything that has happened in my life has been for a good reason.

Doctor Impossible finally guided me to heal myself.

My Spiritual Childhood

I was born in Kfarhilda, a village in Mount Lebanon. My father was a peasant-farmer but also a schoolteacher. He opened the first school in the village, teaching the villagers to read and write under an oak tree after putting the oxen to rest. He loved to read books and to work the land. His culture was inspired by nature. He used to say, "I love the land because it never lies and I hate the hypocrisy of the world."

Kfarhilda lies in a valley of wild nature near a river with a beautiful waterfall. Up in the mountains by my village are the biblical cedars *'which God planted'* and the ancient holy Kadisha Valley. My wild land inspired my childhood with its profound spirituality.

In my childhood I believed that God lived up on top of the mountains and that His spirit filled the whole valley. I found my angels there in the wilderness and they lifted me above all wretchedness. I grew up in the wilderness and the wilderness lived within me. I loved its purity and listened to its songs of beauty. I became a wild rock, refusing to be sculpted and painted by the fashions of modern civilisation.

I lived most of my childhood sitting on the harsh and steep rocks of the valleys, which were full of spirits. I spent my days hugging snakes and sleeping in caves beside wild animals, stroked by black spiders and dark golden

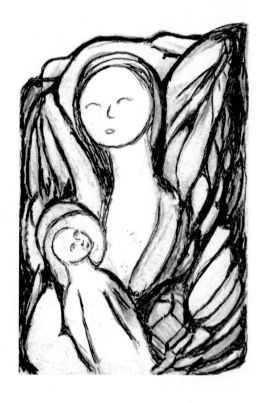

scorpions as they crawled on my head. I followed goats, rabbits and squirrels, dancing with them upon the hills and eating their food.

One cold winter morning the mountains were covered with snow. I walked in the woods praying aloud, absorbed in spiritual ecstasy and unaware of where I was going. Looking around, I found myself in an open field surrounded by a pack of wolves. They were watching me for signs of fear so that they could kill and eat me.

I smiled at the hungry wolves and looked at their beauty. A compassionate wish to feed them burst within me. I wanted to talk to them and give them my body. I felt as if they were the god Ba'al and I was their human sacrifice. I raised my arms like a high priest at the altar and chanted "This is my body, eat it. This is my blood, drink it." They became quiet and still, fallen into a trance. They were enchanted by my spell and no longer preparing to attack. They were stunned and looked at me sideways with their beautiful eyes, leaving me alone to continue my walk in the woods.

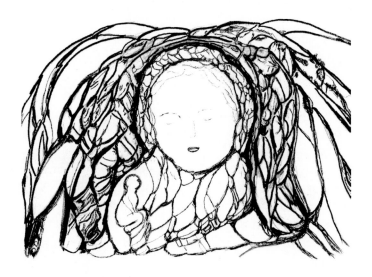

I was also good friends with insects, talking like King Solomon to the ants. One day I was angry at my father after he had beaten me for being different. Nobody was willing to defend me, so I appealed to the ants to help me frustrate my father as he had frustrated me. I invited them to steal all the sugar and grains of wheat which he had collected in bags in our kitchen. They were happy to accept my invitation. I stretched a sweetened thread for my dear ant friends from their holes in the garden to the kitchen. They followed the path I made for them and did their job well, expressing their support for me by invading the kitchen and stealing all the food. I was glad that they had listened to me and taken revenge on my father on my behalf. They were more affectionate to me than he was.

One day I planted a vine tree in a hidden corner of our garden. I went to it nearly every day, giving it my full attention. My passion for my tree helped it to grow fast and produce a beautiful bunch of grapes within a year. I waited hungrily for my fruit to ripen. When the grapes were fully ripe I went to pick them, but was extremely dismayed to find that wasps had already eaten them. Only one grape had survived, which two big red wasps were eating before my eyes! I became furious and decided to send them to prison. I caught them by their wings and put them into a vacuum sealed bottle, not knowing that they would suffocate. I left the bottle under two feet of water in a small pool for several months. In mid-January I went to free them from their watery jail. I took the bottle from the water, opened it, and was astonished to find that they were lifeless.

I was shocked, full of regret and sorrow for having treated them so unjustly. How could I have been so blind as to have committed such a crime? They had the same right as I did to eat my grapes. They were innocent, not knowing they were stealing my fruit; the whole world was their kitchen. How had I allowed myself to kill them? How could I have been so ugly? I took their corpses to pray for them, arranged their funeral, confessed my sinfulness to God and asked the wasp spirits to forgive me.

Suddenly I noticed that their bodies were intact. They had been preserved by the cold vacuum. Great compassion flowed through me, giving me a sense that I could revive them. I placed my warm hands on them and massaged their cold bodies to stimulate their respiratory systems. Within a few minutes they slowly started to move their legs, mouths and wings. After five minutes the two wasps returned to life and were soon able to fly. I felt that my sins were forgiven and love could raise the dead.

I couldn't tell these stories to the local villagers. They wouldn't have understood them and I had to keep what I was doing secret. I was lonely and had no-one with whom to share the beauty of my spiritual life. I wanted my villagers to become interested in my playful world, so I decided to train chickens to perform a special dance for them.

My parents kept a cockerel and six hens in a fenced yard beside the house. One summer morning I awoke to the sound of cackling. Thinking that a fox had upset the hens, I rushed outside to see what was happening and found to my surprise that the chickens were welcoming my mother. She was coming from the field carrying a sheaf of green corn for them. Their cackling sounded like a choir. I thought that hunger could condition any behaviour. If chickens knew how to sing they could also be taught to dance. I would civilise them! I shut them up in their coops without any food. My parents thought I was crazy. I explained my plan to them, but they didn't understand and became angry at me for wanting to carry out such an experiment. I insisted until they yielded and allowed me to proceed.

Drawing a straight white line on the ground, I drove an iron peg into the earth at each end of the line, tied a piece of string between the pegs a few inches higher than the chickens' heads and attached a bit of bread every eighteen inches along the string. I called three of my playmates to join me to form an orchestra. We cut reeds from the river bank to make flutes with them and then rehearsed a tune I'd composed, two of us playing the flutes while the others loudly beat drums.

Everything was now ready so I freed the starving chickens to wander through the garden searching for food. On finding the bits of bread I'd fastened to the string they jumped up to catch them. Squawking tunelessly, they flapped their wings wildly to the rhythm of our music. After two weeks of rehearsal the show was ready to open. The whole village turned out for the premiere of the Great Chicken Dance. As we started to play, the hungry birds rushed out and started marching down the white line. Squawking and flapping, they leapt high into the air where I had previously put the string with their food, even though it was no longer there. Only after the music had stopped were the chickens able to cease their wild and futile dance. At the end I rewarded them with a copious dinner. That is how I trained a dance troupe in my very own fashion. In front of our house I now had a Circus, a Chicken Disco! The village audience laughed at me, thinking that I was ridiculously eccentric! They didn't realise that we can all be conditioned by hunger, just like any chicken.

From childhood I refused the dark side by seeing only the goodness in everyone. I lived through every tear and every smile to nourish my heart with joy. To fulfil my dreams I chose to study medicine to relieve suffering. I did my early medical studies at the American University of Beirut and then went on to university in Cluj, Romania. During the first years of my studies I thought medicine could bring happiness to humanity. Genetics was then entering its high season. I embraced its new approach, hoping one day it would solve many human problems by discovering the gene of human happiness and turning our planet into paradise. I became so excited by this beautiful dream that I wrote and published a book describing my genetic scientific perspective in the form of visionary poetry, which I submitted it as my medical thesis. It was accepted by the examination board and I received my medical diploma in 1983.

Returning to my village, I started to work as a general practitioner. I loved everyone, even those who exploited me and never cared for worldly things, giving up material possessions to remain a free spirit dedicated to healing the sick.

I often loved to walk from my village through the beautiful fields and along paths leading to the mountain tops. One cold March morning I awoke to find the mountains and hills around my village covered with snow. Everything was dressed in white. Trees looked like almonds in flower. The sun was bright and warmed the late winter air. Enjoying the fresh air of the coming spring, I climbed the high rocky cliffs up to the top of a mountain overlooking the deep mystical valley. There I stood in silence, watching the immaculate white of the wilderness after the snowy night.

Hidden amongst the shadows of the great rocks and strange caves, an ancient monastery suddenly caught my eye and drew me towards it. As I entered it to pray and meditate, an old monk appeared. His face shone with the light of humility and serenity. It seemed as if he had emerged out of silence after millennia passed in the monastery caves. I stood perplexed before him. Suddenly he was gone.

I quietly started to visit the monastery, praying for the monk to reappear. Was he a disembodied saint? One day I arrived there in extremely difficult spiritual circumstances. I called out to the Unknown. Suddenly there broke through a light from beyond, revealing the monk's countenance filled with fatherly compassion. I fell on my face and opened my burning heart in tearful confession. As if coming from the empty wilderness of the Universe, a great voice addressed me.

"Listen to the pain! Carry the pain of others. Be the compassionate servant of truth. Open your heart and accept joyfully the frustrations of others.

"Listen to your inner awareness. Embrace the highest human values with your selfless medical compassion.

"Be a servant, carrying the torch of healing and curing the sick. You are neither medical bureaucrat nor scientific robot. You are a gifted man, an artist of life who suffers with every patient and rejoices with them in their healing.

"Be holy in your approach. Light with your love the wick of the lamp of medical science. Guide the sick to their wholeness and carry their burden along the way. Inspire them with the great meaning of life that underlies all suffering.

"Treat the patient as a human being and not a biological machine. Unlock every heart with the key of wisdom and love.

"Cleanse your heart of all worldly addiction, including to yourself. You are not a healer, you are the phoenix in every soul.

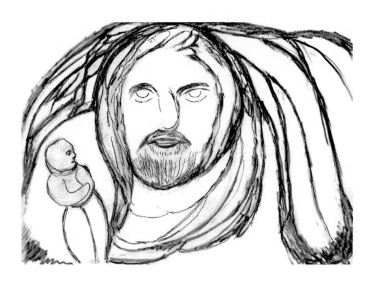

"Be comforted and accept others' greed for you. They may rob you of all your worldly possessions, but they can neither empty you of love nor steal your natural inner happiness.

"Your love will heal many. It will bring miracles of happiness because it has no expectations, no neediness and no fear of truth.

"Continuously instil within yourself the simplicity of inner peace and harmony and always treasure Me in your heart."

But I found it so difficult in my medical work to satisfy everyone, particularly myself. In medical school I learned how to diagnose disease and treat it with drugs and surgery, but it requires more than that to deal with human reality. Does the medicine I studied in medical school give patients what they ask for? Can it do what it promises people or meet their expectations? Everyone would like medicine to solve all their health problems and make them happy.

When I started my practice throughout rural Lebanon in 1984, I had to consider the mind of every patient and listen to their pain and suffering with my entire being. With empathy, I treated the patient as a whole, not just a body, often having to use whatever unconventional approach became available while challenging every fear and anxiety. I risked much by taking full responsibility for patients' lives and sharing their agony, unafraid of any possible consequences. To cure them, I had to retain my medical integrity and human principles in the face of every difficult situation, expanding my medical consciousness to help them, particularly when it seemed impossible. Whenever faced with human suffering I became part of it until I received my healing inspiration. As I spoke with God in my childhood wilderness so I spoke to Him within my patients. Their suffering often provoked my altruistic spirit to seek strength from anywhere to help them. Whenever I treated someone I felt within myself a beautiful world of love and harmony. My challenge was to cure the incurable; the more difficult the medical case, the more compassion and confidence I felt to solve it.

I soon had patients all over Lebanon. My compassion often put me in great danger, but I was prepared to risk everything for the sake of others.

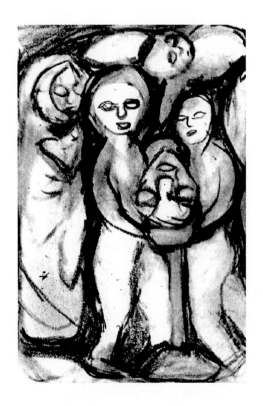

Medical Adventures

One summer afternoon while I was picking grapes in the field near my house a military jeep stopped at the front door. Two armed militiamen rushed towards me, calling out at the top of their voices, "Doctor, Doctor, please come quickly." I hurried towards them to see what the problem was. Behind them stood a woman in tears holding her ten year old son in her lap. "What's the matter?" I asked.

"My son fell to the ground from the roof," she answered. "He's dizzy and can't speak, the right side of his head is swollen and he's vomiting. I don't know what to do. Please help me, Doctor! Save my son!"

We carried the boy to a room on the ground floor of my parents' house and I quickly examined him. His case was of the utmost urgency. His muscles were becoming hypotonic, the pupil of his right eye was slightly enlarged and he was about to lose consciousness. As I examined the child, I saw that his head was severely swollen in the right temporal region and felt that a heavy subdural haemorrhage was occurring. The haematoma was rapidly increasing in size, compressing the brain tissues. By increasing intracranial pressure it would damage the brain, causing cerebral oedema. The boy was in a state of stupor; if the haematoma was left to swell for another half an hour he would have irreversible brain damage and die. The blood collecting under the temporal bone was increasing, pressing further and further on the cortex. The pool of blood building up beneath the boy's skull needed to be removed rapidly. If I were to send him to the nearest hospital in Byblos, more than an hour's drive away, he would die on the way. Heavy artillery shelling had already closed all roads leading to my village. The day before, snipers had shot in the head and killed two young men from a nearby village who had been driving along the road. In an earlier incident two men from my village had been kidnapped from their car at a military checkpoint and their bodies discovered a week later thrown under a bridge.

What could I do for the child under these circumstances? I had just started practising medicine in my village, had no room in my parents' house to use as a clinic and was without medical instruments. But I couldn't abandon the poor boy! How could I shirk my responsibility and tell his mother to take him to the nearest hospital when I knew that he would be dead on arrival?

I was in a dreadful dilemma, with no medical assistant or physician to assist me and share my burden. I looked at the pupils of the poor sweet boy, which were becoming more dilated. His vomiting had stopped, his body was extremely flabby and the swelling of his temporal bone had increased. His case was now critical; he was becoming drowsy and starting to lose consciousness. While his mother was crying and imploring me to do something to help her son, the two gunmen who had brought the boy in their jeep were starting to look very aggressive. Perhaps they were war criminals, hell-bent on theft and murder. They were pressing me in an extremely threatening way to help the boy.

21

I weighed up the situation and told the woman regretfully, "There's nothing I can do to help your son. His case is impossible." Between sobs, she replied "Doctor, help my son! Save his life! Go on, do something; God will lend you a hand!"

The mother's words touched my heart so much that I was almost ready to cry with her. I was in the grip of a deadly dilemma, shaking, hardly able to breathe... I had to drain the blood. The child needed an urgent trepanation! Spotting a hammer and sharp nail in a corner of the room, I seized them, rushing wildly, and suddenly found myself with one hand positioning the nail on the boy's head to hammer it through his skull. A mist obscured my vision. My inner voice called me from The Wilderness, saying, "Go on! Your life is not more important than the boy's. Die with him or live with him!"

I drove the nail through the boy's parietal bone. His blood gushed out, he screamed, his mother wailed and fainted and the two gunmen put their guns to my head, yelling, "You've killed him! You're not a doctor, you are a murderer. We are going to shoot you in the head. Prepare to die!" But I turned round to face the ignorant gunmen with a clear conscience, relieved that I had saved the boy.

"Don't worry, calm down!" I told them quietly. "I have saved this child's life by releasing the pressure of the blood accumulating in his head, which would have damaged his brain. We need to drive quickly to the nearest hospital. The boy now has a chance of arriving there safely. I carried out a quick neurosurgical operation to stop the bleeding. He's still alive and will be OK. I trepanned his skull with a nail because I had no other tools at my disposal, otherwise he would have died. Please listen to me! There'll be plenty of time for you to kill me later. Let's drive quickly to the hospital and on our way we we'll switch to a Red Cross ambulance from one of the military bases to avoid snipers on the road. This is an emergency - we need to leave this very minute!"

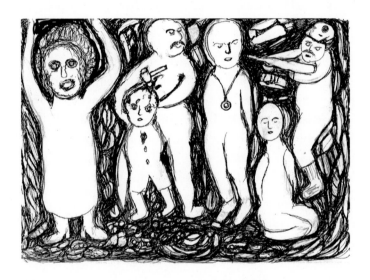

The gunmen and the mother overcame their terrible shock and we all left together with the boy, heedless of the cannon shells exploding around us on the way. Our sole concern was to get him safely to hospital. By the time we got there the injured lad was looking better. Greatly relieved that he had escaped haemorrhagic shock and brain damage, I picked him up, carried him to the emergency ward and summoned the neurosurgeon. He arrived in a few minutes and I told him the whole story. Looking at me strangely while he examined the boy, he must have thought I was some kind of sadistic medical primitive. He scrutinised me and said angrily, "You killed him! You're crazy! I won't take responsibility for helping this child after what you have done to him."

I tried again to explain the situation to my colleague but he refused to listen. I couldn't blame him because our medical texts do not yet recommend home brain surgery with hammer and nail. I looked carefully at the boy, who obviously needed immediate medical attention. Putting my hand on the surgeon's arm I said, "Look here, Doctor, we need to co-operate. If something goes wrong I'll take full responsibility." The neurosurgeon refused to change his mind and looked as if he was trying to escape, so I grabbed his arm tightly and played my last remaining card.

"Listen to me! We must take the boy at once to the emergency clinic before any complications occur. If you don't do as I say the militiamen waiting outside will shoot us." As if to emphasise my words, the two soldiers entered the room looking extremely menacing. When they saw me arguing with the doctor while the boy lay unattended on a hospital trolley they started to shake with rage and pressed the barrels of their guns to our heads. One of them whispered to us in an ice-cold voice, "Save his life or you're both dead men." The surgeon turned as pale as a ghost. In that moment of extreme fear, we smiled at each other and he murmured in a trembling voice, "All right, let's do our best for the boy. We're in God's hands now."

Blood tests showed a mild haemorrhage. A brain scan revealed that the haematoma had been successfully drained by my primitive trepanation and there was no need for further surgery. All the surgeon had to do was to give intravenous corticoid, anti-epileptic and antibiotic drugs for three days. Within a week the child had fully recovered.

I returned to my village feeling relieved and exhausted. Next day at four in the morning I awoke to the sound of knocking. My mother opened the front door and found two men standing outside. "What do you want at this hour?" she said.

"We want your son the doctor to come with us. Our father is dying and before he passes away he would like to see him, not to be treated but to be consoled by being granted his last wish." "Are you sure he's dying?" asked Mother.

"Yes, he's in his seventies and has had every possible medical treatment. His doctor has sent him home to die surrounded by his family. We're now preparing his funeral and have already bought the coffin."

"Why do you really want my son to visit your father?"

"We told you, he's insisting on seeing your son the Doctor before he breathes his last. All we want is for him to come with us now as a goodwill gesture or we'll be blamed."

Mother looked doubtful. "Perhaps what your father really wants is for my son to join him in the grave!"

I overheard the conversation and decided to go to visit the old man. Dressing hurriedly, I took my medical kit with me in case I might need it to help him to die peacefully and went with the two brothers to see their father. Upon entering the house, I saw a crowd sitting around an old person waiting for his death. The moribund patient lay in bed in a state of stupor. His name was Hanna. The people around him told him loudly that I had come to see him, but he gave no response. His sons came closer to see if their father was still conscious and shook him gently, saying, "Hanna, Hanna, the doctor has come to see you."

All of a sudden he awoke from his lethargy, sat up and climbed down from his bed. Everyone thought it was a miracle. Had my appearance brought Hanna back to life? Might I even be able to cure him and prevent his death? Upon examining him, I diagnosed renal insufficiency and cardiac arrhythmia. However serious his case was, I took the view that administering the latest pharmaceutical products to him could save his life and thought that it was worth a try. If worst came to worst and he died under my hands while I was treating him no-one would blame me, since his death at any moment was expected anyway.

I started by giving him a profusion of medical drugs ranging from vitamins, diuretics and cardiac tonics to corticoids, but after half an hour of my sophisticated medical treatment Hanna's heart had almost stopped beating. Could my treatment has caused his cardiac arrest? What happened? I needed to act urgently - perhaps he wasn't completely dead but only in a state of clinical death, in which case I hoped I might be able to bring him back to life.

The watching villagers thought he was about to breathe his last and rushed to call the village priest to administer extreme unction to him. Their Christian Maronite tradition is to have the priest anoint the foreheads of the dying with consecrated oil, praying for God to receive their souls in peace. Without knowing that the villagers had sent for the priest, I struggled to get Hanna out of cardiac arrest by massaging his chest vigorously. Whilst I was absorbed in my attempts to revive him the priest came up behind me, simply trying to do his job, and asked me to stop treating Hanna and leave him in peace so he could bless him before he died. Hanna's heart suddenly started to throb, his pulse returned and his face lost its ghostly pallor, regaining its colour as his limbs became warmer and consciousness returned. His eyes began to open.

The priest impetuously shoved me out of his way to put the oil of unction on Hanna's brow. The sight of his dark

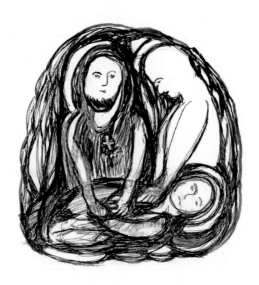

figure looming over Hanna and praying for his death could have produced a lethal psychological impact on such an old man, and I didn't want anyone interfering at such a critical moment. Clearly seeing Hanna coming back to life, I totally rejected any idea that he might be dead or anyone waiting to bury him.

Encouraged by the villagers, the priest pressed me to leave the old man to go in peace to his Father in heaven. "Stop!" I exclaimed, as he put his hand on the perfusion glucose bag to tear it away. I simply couldn't allow him to bless Hanna's death and knocked him to the floor, shouting, "Father, it's my turn now, not yours! When you hear the bell toll you can come back to finish your job."

Angry and astonished at my violent reaction towards the priest, everyone was ready to attack me to defend his holiness, but as soon as they realised Hanna had regained consciousness they remained frozen and stupefied. The crowd left the house in silence and went home.

Hanna was completely healed and lived on for another fifteen years.

On the way back to my house I began to wonder whether my compassion was driving me beyond the limit. Thank God for bringing Hanna back to life! For him to have died after I'd knocked down the priest would have been unbearable for me, and my reputation would probably have been destroyed. Instead, it continued to grow. My home clinic in Kfarhilda started to be besieged by continuous hordes of patients coming from all the surrounding towns and villages. For days and nights I hardly slept a wink. My mother became was so concerned about my health that she was always trying to stop patients coming to wake me up while I was trying to sleep.

One day a car stopped in front of my house from which two young men emerged shouting, "Doctor! Doctor! Come quickly, Kareemy the wife of Khalil is dying." I hurried to see what the matter was. When I arrived at her house it was crowded with villagers who had heard sounds of quarrelling and were there to find out what was happening.

Kareemy lay groaning in bed. I examined her and found that her blood pressure was extremely high. She was at great risk of having a cerebro-vascular accident (a stroke) and I knew I had to get her blood pressure down quickly. I gave her injections of hypotensive drugs and diuretics, but to no avail. Her blood pressure remained the same. I administered even larger doses but it still wouldn't drop. Her face and body looked extremely tense, as if she had suffered a nervous shock induced by fear and anxiety, so I examined her more carefully.

While I was checking her blood pressure, Khalil appeared from behind me like a ghost, his eyes burning red with anger. Hovering over his wife like a hawk, he started screaming, "Kareemy, you careless woman, I'll kill you! Haha! You let the cow graze on our potato plants! The whole year's crop is lost. Now I'm going to finish you off for good!" As Khalil yelled at her Kareemy's blood pressure shot up to 240mm Hg. The right side of her face and tongue started to droop and her speech became slurred, but he still went on threatening her. Kareemy's terror of her husband's cruelty was inducing a stroke and I knew I had to act fast to eliminate the stress of fear. I was so frustrated by the ineffectiveness of my pharmaceuticals and infuriated by Khalil's continuing provocation. Crazy with anger, he suddenly tried to push me out of his way, leaving Kareemy to die. I had to do something to cast out the evil, so out of compassion for her and with all my strength I shoved him out of the door. He fell heavily to the floor and I admonished him, "If you go on behaving like this with your wife you'll kill her and be responsible for her death. You should respect and love her. She is a wonderful woman."

Everyone burst out laughing at what had happened and Khalil fled the house in fear. As I looked at Kareemy she appeared relaxed, evidently now free of Khalil's stress and no longer terrorised by him. Her fear had left her and she could breathe better, a smile returning to her face. I measured her blood pressure, which had dropped to 160 mm Hg, close to normal.

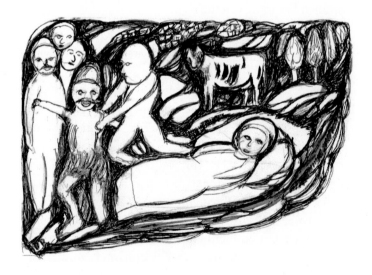

"You're all right now," I told her. "Just take pills every day to avoid any rise in your blood pressure and remember not to let the cow graze on your potatoes and cabbages."

Tired and drained of energy, I started to ponder over the many strange and difficult situations I was getting myself into. How on earth had my aggressive and out of order therapeutic approach not ended up getting me killed? What bizarre kind of doctor was I, anyway? Why did I have to behave so madly to rescue my patients' lives, banging nails into heads, knocking down priests and kicking people out of their houses? I was so wild and uncontrollable, and never gave a damn whether or not my weird behaviour got me into trouble. I'd been very lucky to stay alive after all my adventures; my guardian angel must have been working overtime to protect me.

By now, after all I'd gone through, I began to feel brave enough to risk everything to go far beyond the boundaries of medicine. Starting to feel able to overcome anything and everything that might hinder me from helping my patients, I saw the need for different approaches and better ways to treat them, rather than the somewhat inefficient traditional ones I had become used to. I continued my medical adventures...

Fifty-year-old Mr X had suffered from back pain for over ten years and tried everything to cure it. Painkillers, anti-inflammatory drugs, acupuncture, physiotherapy, spiritual healing, homeopathy, osteopathy and sympathy: in the end nothing worked and the pain got worse. In time, I became Mr X's friend and family doctor. With great confidence, he started to believe that I was the only doctor in the world who would be able to cure his back pain. He asked me to find or invent any therapeutic approach which might help him. I was eager to discover a remedy for him. But how? He'd already tried everything under the sun. All the clever sciences had failed to solve his problem. Where on earth could I find the answer to his dilemma? Maybe I was foolish, even crazy to think this way. But then again, X's case might need a fool, a fool with a solution.

Faeki, an old peasant who lived in my village, came to my mind. Perhaps he had the answer. People called him the village fool; he had never been to school and couldn't even sign his name, but he was wise. In his own way he understood everything. He was so natural and simple he could intuitively answer any question. Faeki was my friend. His heart was always open to me. He knew how to listen. Whenever I needed advice he told me what to do! I visited him one day after finishing my hard work in the hospital. I felt that he would inspire me with his naive simplicity and intuitive wisdom and answer my impossible question.

"Faeki, how can I cure chronic back pain? I have a patient no-one has been able to help. What should I do?" He chuckled and replied, "Teach him to rub his back with hot sand like a donkey." I laughed and said, "The donkey is the most stupid animal. How can I learn anything from it?"

"No, donkeys are the greatest scientists ever born. You need to trust their wisdom completely. Listen and I'll tell you a true donkey story. You'll see how wise they are."

"OK, go on, Faeki," I replied.

"High up in the mountains, near the Valley of Ghosts, strange things were happening. The weather was very unusual. It often rained there in summertime but nowhere else.

"An old woman lived there called 'Magic Woman' because only she always knew when it was going to rain. She could foretell bad weather when no-one else could."

"Faeki," I interrupted, "what is all this nonsense about? What does your story about donkeys, rain, old women and magic have to do with curing back pain?"

Faeki tapped my shoulder hard and frowned. "Young man," he said, "don't be so impatient! Slow down and listen. Stop interrupting me and let me finish my story." I shut my mouth, emptied my head and sat quietly before wise old Faeki. I felt that he was taking me back to the days of my childhood, when I loved visiting his cottage and listening to his fairy tales. He went on with his tale.

"Scientists wanted to study the strange weather, so they decided to spend a few days up in the mountains. They settled down next to the old woman's cottage and began to set up their apparatus. She soon came up and warned them not to stay in their tents that night, but instead to come into her cottage to sleep. When they asked her why, she told them there would be a heavy storm that night which would put them in danger. It was a beautiful sunny day and the sky was clear and cloudless. The scientists looked in disbelief at the old woman and laughed at her. They read their instruments and told her that the weather would stay fine.

'Don't worry about us,' they said, 'we'll be OK. It won't rain.'

'Listen to me carefully, young men! I am warning you: a storm is coming tonight. Come with me now into the safety of my cottage. Come, before I close the door and windows to protect myself from the terrible storm.' The scientists thought that she was cuckoo and ignored her.

"After midnight, while they were all fast asleep, a gale blew down from the mountain. Heavy rain flooded down and washed away their tents. Desperate to escape, they rushed to the woman's cottage door and hammered on it, shouting, 'We're your scientist friends. We apologise! Please let us in before we all drown!'

"The old lady felt sorry for them, so she opened the door and let them in. She welcomed them, dried their wet clothes, gave them all a cup of hot tea and prepared beds for them.

"At ten in the morning the scientists awoke from their heavy sleep. The wind had calmed, the sky was clear and the sun shone bright. The Valley of Ghosts glistened with dripping greenery. With nothing left for them to do all day, the clever men sat sheepishly at the breakfast table with Magic Woman and started to ask her lots of silly questions.

'Dear lady, thank you for your help and hospitality. Would you please reveal to us how you knew that there would be a storm last night? We would be very grateful if you could share your secret with us.' The old lady laughed and answered, 'I shall be delighted to introduce you to my great master, from whom I have learned advanced meteorology. If he likes you, with one look from him you'll be enlightened. I can guarantee that he will reveal to you his General Theory.'

'Who is he? Where is he?' asked the scientists. 'Please give us a brief introduction to his theory so we will be better prepared to understand such a great genius! Just think how this wonderful knowledge will serve science and benefit humanity.'

'Don't be in such a hurry, my dear children. Finish your cup of tea and then we'll go to meet my teacher.' They drank their tea quickly and made for the door. To their surprise, the old woman led them to a small stable.

'Wait here a moment,' she said. She went into the stable and came out leading a squint-eyed old donkey on a rope. Looking with concern at the bewildered scientists, she took a deep breath and spoke. 'You look very tired. You didn't sleep a wink last night.'

'Don't worry about us, we're fine,' they replied impatiently. 'Hurry up and introduce us to your great teacher; we want him to collaborate with us. We're men of science and can't afford to waste time.' The old woman gave them a penetrating look.

'Very well,' she replied, 'you told me you wanted a basic introduction to my master's teachings. Listen carefully - I am about to reveal his secret to you!' The whole group fell silent and bowed their heads with bated breath as Magic Woman started to speak.

'When the weather is going to be stormy with heavy rain, my donkey senses danger and refuses to stay outside. He brays continuously until I bring him to the stable. Yesterday he shook his ears and tail to tell me that a strong storm was coming. I listened to him with a humble heart because I understand him. You are different. You ignored me yesterday because your scientific knowledge has blinded you. This donkey is my great teacher. He understands the world better than I do. If you really want to know about nature ask my donkey.' They all guffawed at her outrageous advice!

"Shaking her head, she turned to the donkey and whispered in his ear. He looked briefly at the scientists with his squinty eye and walked back to his stable."

I laughed, but couldn't help feeling that Faeki was telling me the story to make fun of me and was jeering at my educated scientific mind. But what can one expect from a fool? He is free to say whatever comes into his mind, with no responsibility and nothing to lose. The real fool was me for having taken him seriously.

Raging inside, I smiled politely at Faeki and thanked him for his charming donkey tale. In a smooth voice I said, "My dear Faeki, are you telling me to go and ask some donkey to teach me how to cure chronic back pain? Maybe you are. Is it possible that after so many years of medical practice I'm still too stupid to cure back pain? Yes, you have forced me to acknowledge my scientific stupidity which brought me here. You are absolutely right, Faeki. Thank you so much!" Faeki ignored my sarcasm and nodded quietly. "Yes," he replied, "I want you to do exactly that. The true doctor who is able to learn medicine even from donkeys."

I stood up stiffly, staring at Faeki, and suddenly all my frustrations exploded. I threw back my head, screwed up my eyes and leapt into the air, punching the sky and screaming, "I am going immediately to smash the back of the first donkey I meet! I shall observe the injured donkey carefully to see whether and how he can heal himself and if he can and if I can learn some new technique from him with which I might perhaps be able to benefit my patients, then, and only then, Faeki, will you have been proved right!"

Maybe I needed to smash my own thick head and not some poor old donkey. Faeki was no fool, his words were true and had been given through him in a spirit of high wisdom as a personal message to me.

In November 1985 I was picking olives in the mountain groves and had filled two sacks. I tied them to my donkey's back to bring them home. On the way, he stumbled on the rugged path and collapsed. He couldn't get up, so I untied the ropes and removed the sacks of olives, allowing him to relax himself. Faeki's story came to my mind. What would the donkey do?

"My dear donkey, if you can really heal your own back please show me how now!" I quietly asked, feeling great sympathy for him.

As soon as he had been released from his burden he wobbled back into the field and found a heap of soft, hot sand to lie on. He stretched out his body on the sand, flexed his legs and rolled over several times until his back straightened and his vertebral muscles were loosened. After his self-massage, the donkey walked over to a tree and rubbed his back against it. He shook the sand from his body, came up to me and pressed himself against my hands. He clearly wanted me to give him a pain-relieving massage, so I did as he asked. His back pain disappeared and he was soon able to carry the olives home.

This experience inspired me to create a completely new way to manipulate deep fascial pain receptors, triggering the self-correcting function of muscle groups. I was astonished to see how my donkey not only knew exactly which subtle energy centres needed stimulation but was even able to teach me this new healing skill. Thank

God that my childhood wilderness gave me the gift of communication with animals.

I was impatient to try out my new method on Mr. X, so I went to explain my discovery to him. He got very excited and asked me to try it out on him immediately. I applied the Donkey Technique to him and within half an hour it had produced miraculous results, completely curing his chronic back problem. This was the first time I had used only my hands in practising medicine. From then on I started to understand it in unusual new ways. I observed that when we force our vertebral back muscles beyond their capacity their fibres contract, become densely compacted

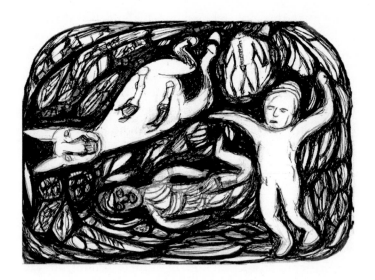

and unable to relax. They eventually become atrophied, restrict vertebral movement and cause pain. The donkey knew intuitively how to heal himself. He lay down on hot sand to allow the heat to warm and relax his muscles, then he gradually stretched them with exercise and afterwards rubbed the remaining contracted muscle fibres on a tree and against my hands.

I noticed how the donkey looked at me with sweet eyes full of empathy when he was in pain. He was silently asking me for help, as if telling me to use my fingers to press his painful tissues to regulate the endomysium tissue surrounding the muscle fibres and stimulate the neuromuscular junctions. Did he know that I was a doctor? Whether or not he did isn't very important, but I am sure of one thing: the medical revolution he inspired in me confirmed that he himself truly was a great doctor.

In medical school, I was taught that in cases of muscular pain I should first use anti-inflammatories to reduce the inflammation and then apply physiotherapy. In cases like the donkey's such medical protocols are inappropriate because the problem is biomechanical. My view is that in cases where a muscular problem is due to a functional disorder in the biomechanics of the muscles, the treatment should be based not only on a chemical pharmaceutical approach but also on a biomechanical one. The effort consumed by our back muscles is called work capacity, which is related to the weight of the human body and the muscular force applied over time. When the effort is excessive and stress exceeds the resistance limit the muscles become spastic. If the spasm persists then the muscular tissue becomes chronically inflamed, leading in time to atrophy, calcification, sclerosis and degeneration.

My medical adventure with my donkey opened the way for me to see neuro-osteo-muscular medicine as a new biomechanical science.

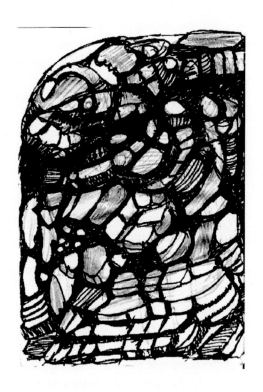

Healing Reflections

It was Summer, 1987. The story about how I had cured Mr X simply with my hands spread like wildfire. An elderly Lebanese-Argentine gentleman who had retired to his native village ten miles away heard the news and invited me to visit him in his home. He wanted me to examine him, diagnose his illness and see whether I could help him. Twenty years earlier he had been cured of laryngeal cancer.

Upon entering his house I noticed that his walk was chaotic and bizarre. He had difficulty moving without supporting himself against a wall. His left leg appeared rigid, was about four inches shorter than the other and he couldn't flex his toes. Struggling hard, he dragged himself along as he came to greet me. I saw how he overcame all obstacles in his way, refusing to become completely disabled. His suffering had started twenty-five years earlier. He visited many clinics all over the world to no avail and no one knew what the matter was with him. But he hadn't lost hope and was full of confidence and love of life. I pondered over his problem for a few minutes and thought at first that it would be very difficult for me to treat his case. I apologised for being unable to do anything for him. Seeing my frustration at my incapacity to help him, he gently invited me to join him for a coffee. I felt his compassion and started to listen. Out of desperation I started to pray silently.

"O Lord, You who healed the sick, help me in this difficult situation. I, who left everything in life to follow in Your steps, am helpless if You do not direct me! O Lord, You who love me, I implore You to guide me in my medical practice. I seek neither money nor glory. I need Your mercy and Your help to heal the sick. Amen!"

Two minutes after my silent prayer the man suddenly said, "Doctor, you haven't examined me or even touched me. How can you judge my case without a proper examination?" "OK," I replied, "you're right. I'll examine you thoroughly and will try physical therapy on the weak muscles. Then we'll see."

He undressed and lay down on his bed. I put my hand on his sacral region and pressed it hard with my thumb. His problem had to lie somewhere in the muscular coxofemoral reigion towards the greater sciatic foramen. Examining the area, I felt through palpation how the musculature had become chronically contracted, trapping and almost paralysing the sciatic nerve. The muscles had atrophied around the head of the femur, shortening the patient's leg and making him unable to extend it. I applied my hands to soften the chronically contracted area and then stretched the atrophied leg, releasing the trapped sciatic nerve.

The patient immediately felt that something immense had happened to him. He stood up from his bed in an explosion of joy, looked at me stupefied and thrilled and cried, "Doctor, see how my heel can now touch the floor! I haven't been able to do that for the past twenty years. It's a miracle! I feel and see that my left leg is not short any more." It was hard for me to understand what was going on and how it was possible that he had improved so

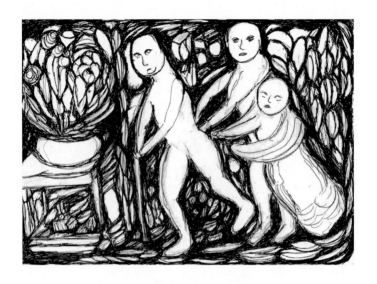

quickly just from my touch. It seemed as if a miracle had happened. How great! I felt wonderful and realised that God was with me.

"Thank you, my Lord! For twenty-five years this man from Argentina looked everywhere for a cure but no-one could help him. Now You have seen fit to heal him through me. Thank you!"

I returned home feeling gratitude that I had found my true path in life. I continued the treatment sessions with my patient until he was completely cured and could walk normally. I was so happy that the Argentine man was healed, and continued along my way more confident in my ability to help others suffering from neuromuscular problems. I felt the healing angel Raphael accompanying me everywhere I went.

Mariam, a poor shepherd's wife from Byblos, heard how I had cured a slipped disc. She had been confined to her bed for six months with a severe discopathy and was desperate for my help.

I went to treat her in her home. I examined Mariam and found that her leg muscles were weak and atrophied. The reflexes of her knees and heels were feeble. At first I felt I could do nothing for her, but something kept pushing me not to give up. I applied vigorous massage, which she found very painful. After enduring several sessions of my physical therapy she couldn't see any improvement. Believing that my treatment had failed, I decided to apply even tougher therapy and started to disentangle the compacted muscle fibres of her legs, just as my grandfather used to beat an old woollen mattress with a stick to recover its elasticity.

After one month, I was happy to find that Mariam's leg muscles were finally working properly again and the hernia in her disc seemed to have disappeared. I ordered her to get out of bed and run up and down the stairs, which she did with ease. Although she appeared fully recovered, I still didn't quite understand how it had happened and wondered why my weird therapy had been so effective. I was shocked. Had her cure happened by itself spontaneously? Was it I who had healed her? Hoping that from Mariam's case I could further develop my new approach to neuromuscular and osteo-articular disorders, I asked her to describe for me how she might have been cured.

She looked at me cautiously. Drawing a deep breath, she closed her eyes and relaxed. A strange light shone from her face as she spoke.

"After you left me last night, I saw how hard you were struggling to cure me and felt your frustration, so I prayed to St. Charbel to help you. After I went to sleep, someone came and shook my shoulder, saying, 'Mariam, Mariam, don't be afraid, I am St. Charbel. Wake up, go and tell your family you are healed.' I woke up and found I was able to move and get up from my bed. I walked round my room shouting with joy and went to kneel in thanks before the icon of St. Charbel. My husband and three children heard the noise and rushed in to see what was going on. I told them all about St. Charbel's miracle and we tearfully embraced each other."

My elaborate scheme to advance the science of medicine went up in smoke. My tongue stuck to the roof of my mouth. I gulped several times and finally managed to blurt out a complete sentence. "Mariam... keep praying to St Charbel. He obviously listens to you!"

Later that year another woman from Byblos who knew about Mariam's 'miracle' invited me to visit her. She wanted me to help her daughter Mary, who suffered from leg and back pain. Mary was unable to walk and had been diagnosed with L4-L5 disc hernia. Neurosurgeons and orthopaedists advised her to have an urgent laminectomy before she became completely paralysed. I knew Mary's case would be very difficult, but after twenty minutes of discussion with her I suddenly felt confident that I could help. As soon as I started to examine her I felt waves of pleasant energy flowing through me and saw my hands moving spontaneously by themselves to her affected areas as if they were being guided. My mind became empty and I felt as if I was in another world.

I opened my eyes and suddenly noticed Mary's mother sitting motionless and gazing at me with deep reverence. Why was she looking at me like that? What was on her mind? What did she see? I smiled at her respectfully and said, "Madam, don't worry about your daughter. She'll be fine."

Raising her hands towards the sky she answered, "I'm not worried about my daughter. I'm sure she will be cured." Tears fell from her eyes and she crossed herself.

"My dear lady, your daughter Mary will soon walk and within two weeks she'll be fully recovered," I replied.

"Yes, God has sent you to heal my daughter."

"There is something unusual about the way you are looking at me," I said. "Do you mind if I ask you what it is?"

At first she was reluctant to answer but, once she felt sure that I was open-minded, she then replied, "My dear doctor, I'll tell you everything after you have finished treating my daughter."

I examined Mary's back and noticed that the paravertebral muscles at L4-L5 were contracted and cramping the disc space. They had compressed the roots of the right sciatic nerve and the gelatin of her vertebral discs, causing a prolapse with consequential leg pain and paralysis. Following my diagnosis, I pressed with my thumb on the contracted muscles by L3-L4-L5, relaxing and stretching them until the nerve was released and no longer trapped. The vertebral

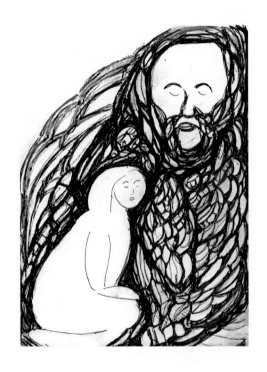

spaces opened and the bulged gelatinous nucleus of the disc returned to normal. After half an hour I examined her to see if my treatment had worked. All the pain in Mary's legs had disappeared. She could move freely and was able to bend down to touch the floor. Her back became straight and flexible and her disc hernia had vanished. I told her to stay in bed for ten days without moving her spine, after which she would be completely recovered.

Several days later I went to visit Mary, but she had left home that morning to visit a monastery. Her mother was glad to see me and offered me coffee. I knew that she was ready to tell me something important.

"The night before you came here to visit Mary I prayed to St. Charbel to heal her. As I slept I dreamed I was walking down an ancient road between old oak trees towards his church. Along the way I met my doctor brother. He asked me why I looked so sad and lonely. I told him that Mary was in great pain and unable to walk. He shook his head and said nothing. As we talked, a strange person suddenly appeared from nowhere before me and said, 'Take this remedy to your daughter.' He held out his hands towards me, joined as if in prayer. He opened them to offer me something but I could see nothing. They were empty. Next morning when my son awoke from sleep he told me he'd heard that you were a good doctor who could help my daughter. We agreed to consult you immediately. As soon as you came through our front door, I recognised you were the same strange man I'd seen in my dream."

From village to village, from town to town and from city to city I drove non-stop to visit my patients in their homes. I continuously had to cross military check points and sometimes had to go through areas where fighting had broken out. I was getting exhausted by the pressure of my situation and decided to open a clinic in Beirut. I found a suitable place in East Beirut with three rooms and a big reception area, where I could manage several patients at the same time.

Early one morning, Alliyah and her son Mohammad walked into my new Beirut clinic to see me. My secretary told her she had to make an appointment, but Aliyah insisted on seeing me immediately because her son needed my urgent help before he became completely paralysed. She had been in such a hurry that she hadn't been able to make an appointment, was financially unprepared and had no money. She fell to her knees in tears, saying that her beautiful young son didn't deserve all the pain he was going through and that I had to help him. She begged my secretary to allow her to see me and kept crying that Allah had sent them. She wailed and wailed.

My secretary didn't know how to deal with Alliyah and tried to ignore her, but it was completely impossible, so she asked her to leave. Alliyah started to beat her breast, pleading with Allah to grant me power, prosperity and long life, and to put His hand onto Mohammad with mine to heal him.

I heard the row going on from my clinic's emergency room where I was treating a war-wounded patient to stop his bleeding. I could hear every word Alliyah was saying through the door and felt very frustrated. I knew that she wanted me to leave everything and go to help Mohammad immediately. But how could I? Should I leave my patient bleeding and go instead to care for Mohammad? Well, my nurse could always treat his wounds, instead of me.

Alliyah went on and on, talking loudly about how Allah would heal her son, and how I was obliged to come immediatly for Him to do His work, so I hurried to treat Mohammad. As I entered my reception room, Alliyah started to calm down.

Her son's back was badly twisted, with numbness and severe pain in his legs. Pressure on his L3-L4-L5-S1 vertebrae was preventing him from standing up or walking properly. Orthopaedic surgeons had recommended an urgent operation to prevent compression of his spinal cord and save him from paralysis. The operation carried a high risk and had only a 10% chance of success.

Alliyah left me to work on him and went out to the corridor, where she took out a small carpet from her handbag, laid it on the floor and started to pray. I continued to examine Mohammad and then applied my hands to his back, relieving the pressure on his spinal cord. Alliyah finished her prayers and came back into the room. She started to tell me how blessed she was and how Allah had guided her son Mohammad to me.

"Last night I went to sleep so frustrated, not knowing the best way to help my son. I woke up at dawn as the muezzins started to recite the call to prayer. Soon I heard someone knocking on my door. It was my neighbour, Sheikh Mustafa. He had heard about you and believed that you could help my son. He woke up early and came to tell me not to take my son Mohammad for surgery, but instead to bring him immediately to you." I was so absorbed in treating Mohammad that I hardly heard a word she said and just replied, "If Allah wills."

"Insha'Allah," she responded. I continued to work on Mohammad's back while Alliyah went on talking and talking. She obviously believed that her words would help me to serve her son better and started to tell me a story.

A barren woman wanted a child. She went to Moses and asked him to speak with Allah to find out whether or not she would become pregnant. Moses posed her question to Allah, who replied that she would not. When the woman heard the news she said "Allah kareem" (God is generous). She soon became pregnant and went back to Moses, asking him to find out whether her pregnancy was contrary to Allah's will. Moses returned to the mountain to ask Him why He had changed His mind.

Allah replied, "Moses, when I said she would have no child, she called Me generous. So how can I not be generous?"

While Alliyah was telling me her story, Mohammad had been crying in agony as I stretched and relaxed his spastic muscles. I hoped that she would tell me more; her magical tales might help me to tranquillise her son's pain. But as soon as she had finished her story, Mohammad calmed down. His tense face started to relax, his back looked straighter and his leg mobility had improved. I asked him to try to walk and to tell me whether he still felt any pain or had any difficulty in moving. Suddenly he jumped to his feet, walked perfectly and began to skip and dance for joy. He was completely healed.

I turned to Alliyah and said "Allah Kareem."

One summer afternoon I wanted to escape from the unbearably hot weather in Beirut, so I drove up to the mountains to visit a young lady friend. As I walked through her door she rushed up to me and said excitedly, "You have come just in time! I've spent the last ten days looking for you. You're always appearing unexpectedly and then disappearing without leaving a trace. We need your help! Come with me to help our best friend Julia. She is in terrible pain."

We went together to the mountain village where Julia and her family lived their simple lives. Their house was filled with visiting peasants and shepherds. When Julia's parents saw me in their house they got very excited and could hardly believe that it was really me. They were so happy that they started to cry.

"Julia is in agony! She's waiting for you in her room," said her mother. "We've been praying to St. Elijah to find you, but you never came. Thank God you're here now. Her right hand is already paralysed. The doctors said there was nothing they could do to save it. If you had arrived in time you could still have cured her. Go and see Julia, she is in bed. Please go by yourself, I can't stand to see my daughter suffering."

As I entered Julia's room I saw her lying in bed moaning. She was in a lot of c pain and her face was pale. Her eyes were closed, her hands extended and she was praying in a low voice for St. Elijah to fetch me to help her. Suddenly she saw me standing by her bedside, but could not believe her eyes and thought she was dreaming. I touched her shoulder gently and then she knew that it was me and could only be me. Smiling joyfully, she cried, "Elijah! Elijah has brought you to me!" Her prayers had been answered.

I quickly started to touch the pain around her neck, shoulders, hand and fingers, massaging her spastic muscles to relax them. Then I pressed my thumbs around her cervical discs C5-C7 to release the contracted tendons pressing upon her brachial plexus until the median nerve was decompressed and the pain relieved. Julia's paralysed hand began to move and within a few minutes it had fully recovered. All was again normal. I was astonished to see how quickly she had been cured. How was it possible? It looked as if St. Elijah had done his job really well.

"Julia, rise from your bed and walk," I commanded her. "Julia, a miracle has happened to you!" She moved her shoulder and hand freely without pain, jumped out of bed and started to dance exuberantly around the room. My heart danced joyfully with her.

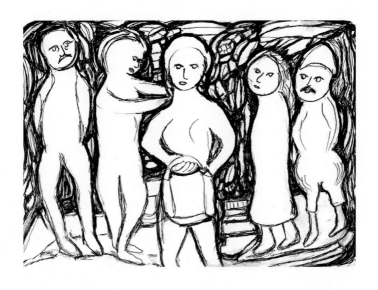

I saw a plastic container full of water in the corner weighing about twenty kilos. I ordered Julia to lift it with the hand that had been paralysed.

"Julia, you are fully cured. Lift this jar with your right hand. Now you can. Its strength has returned. It is no longer paralysed!"

"How can I lift it? Impossible! I can't do it," she cried.

"Julia, it's wonderful how you can raise your hand freely above your head with no pain. It's amazing! Before you couldn't, but now you can. Trust me and do as I ask. Please don't talk, just lift the container."

She grasped the container handle with her right hand and stared at me, exclaiming, "I can't do it, I can't, it's impossible."

"Yes you can. I've fixed your hand and I'm sure you can lift the container. Please don't disappoint me because I believe in you. You are powerful. You can do it. You are a special woman and now you will do it."

Julia picked up the heavy container, lifted it confidently to her breast, put it down and fell to her knees crying out for joy. Her mother and all the neighbours and villagers rushed in to find out what was happening. When they saw how she had been miraculously healed they stood dumbfounded. Without uttering a word, Julia suddenly rushed from the house, leaving me behind with her mother. She didn't return home all day.

What had happened? I had no clue, it was so bizarre. Why had Julia left the house with no goodbye or thank you? Was this to be my reward for all the wonderful work I had performed on her? Had she gone mad from the sudden shock of her instant healing? I started to worry - I don't want people to be so impressed by me that they go insane. I need to be careful not to unbalance my patients' minds while curing their bodies!

Later on, I discovered that Julia had rushed to the church of St. Elijah to thank him instead of me and to offer him a grateful donation for having healed her. I got nothing!

Many in Lebanon were amazed to see how I could cure their serious health problems and quickly relieve their suffering using only my hands. They thought that I performed miracles and was a divinely-gifted doctor, almost like some kind of saint. It was impossible to persuade them otherwise or to explain my healing work using conventional logic, so to avoid endless debate I had to accept their viewpoint. Even I myself was perplexed to see how my hands could produce such extraordinary healing. With no way to understand how it had occurred, my medical mind was baffled and I began to have professional doubts, starting to believe that a healing power from above and beyond apparent reality might really be working through me. I was in conflict within myself: part of my mind was conditioned by sceptical, pragmatic medical thinking, couldn't find a scientific explanation for my healing reality and believed it was all fake; the other part, seeing that my unorthodox medical approach produced fantastic results, readily accepted it, feeling obliged to interpret my healings as paranormal events manifesting through me, at least until I could find a rational explanation for them which would satisfy everyone, regardless of their personal viewpoint.

I had somehow to resolve my conflict. I started to ask myself whether I was really a healer disguised as a doctor with God-given skill. I felt lost and sounded like a delirious mystic.

But how could I possibly believe that my healing gift came from God when I knew how easily I was attracted to the pleasures of worldly indulgence? If I truly had such a splendid gift from God, surely I had a duty to protect and cultivate it by pleasing Him. I wanted Him to be glad and proud that He had given me His Gift. Why not follow His discipline rather than my personal desires? Wouldn't He be jealous and become enraged if I paid more attention to worldly matters than to Him? I certainly didn't want to do anything that might irritate Him. Why take the risk of enjoying so much fun in my life that God would be obliged to disown and abandon me, cutting me off from His healing power?

I felt clueless and directionless. Who or what was manifesting through me? I started to question everything, feeling when I was in a bad mood that demons were manipulating me and when in a good mood angels were guiding me. I was caught and consumed by a conflict of opposites, between God and the Devil. I became wretched, lost between illusion and belief, groping in the dark for my truth, feeling betrayed and deluded. My whole medical foundation had collapsed. I needed help, a guiding inspiration from somewhere. Was there really a spiritual power behind my medical work which had chosen me to perform healing miracles? Should I abandon the world in order for God not to abandon me? Might there possibly be some way for me to become truly spiritual so as to have the divine right to perform my healing miracles? If one day I was able to explain my healings rationally would my dilemma be resolved? Until that day, I had seriously to take into consideration the probability that my healings were the result of a divine gift. I was obliged to believe that God might well be doing his work through me and therefore absolutely had to follow His Will and Discipline.

Yes, that was it! I needed to liberate myself from worldly matters to become purified and peaceful within before it was too late, or God would almost certainly fly into a rage at me and confiscate my healing powers.

And if my gift didn't come from my Lord, nothing would be lost. A bit of fasting never hurt anybody!

I decided to appeal for guidance from a certain gentleman answering to the name of Nuhurianu, an ancient enlightened sage of deep insight whom I used to visit in secret whenever I was in turmoil and losing touch with reality. He understood me perfectly and always assuaged my chaotic moods. I needed his advice, whatever it might turn out to be.

I woke up at the crack of dawn and crept unobserved to share my concerns with my Master. As soon as we met I opened my heart to him, feeling like a little child, and asked him what I had to do to protect my gift. As he listened to me silently, I saw light starting to appear on his face. He rose to his feet, took my hand and told me firmly that I had to learn to practice austerity.

"Yes," I replied, "I agree with you, Master Nuhurianu, but you need to understand that I was born a sensual being. It will be very hard for me to live without worldly desires and pleasures. I don't want to deprive myself of the things I most enjoy - I'm only human!"

He took a deep breath and remained silent for a moment, then walked away, came back, gazed directly into my eyes and started to admonish me.

"My dear son! You must learn to understand that your healing gift will be increased tremendously once you are no longer so attracted to your worldly desires and pleasures. You must live a spiritual life and learn the art of self-mortification, which will greatly help you in your vocation and heighten your humanistic spirit."

"Yes, Master," I replied, "I'm immensely grateful for your helpful words. I will try my best to do exactly as you say."

"Wonderful, excellent, good Boy! It is so beautiful that you are willing to listen to me. I am delighted to hear you intend to follow my advice. Surely now you will never be lost!"

"Master, I need to ask you a rather delicate question. May I please have your permission?"

"Yes, of course you may, my dear boy."

"I have a confession to make to you. I often get a powerful sensual attraction to women. Do you think that sexual indulgence might affect my healing power? I don't want to lose either my pleasurable life or my healing gift. What should I do?"

He roared with laughter. "It's very easy! I have a simple and effective ancient practice for you which I can thoroughly recommend. You've earned it!"

"How wonderful, Master! I can't wait to hear what it is."

"Take a whip with you wherever you go. Whenever you are troubled by sexual thoughts, flog yourself until your heart is cleansed."

"Master, I will do my best to obey your instructions," I replied. "Thank you so much for your great help. But where should I begin? Do you seriously mean to say that I should actually <u>beat</u> myself? "

He looked at me sternly with a little smile playing round his lips and then he handed me a book, saying, "Here is our ancient traditional wisdom. Kindly don't make fun of it!" It was an old leather-bound volume called *A History of the Rod*, written in the reign of Queen Victoria by an English clergyman named the Rev. William M. Cooper. "Take this book home with you and study it carefully," he commanded me. "It contains much valuable information which I'm confident you will find very helpful."

I was fascinated by the book. It was all about flagellation through the ages. At the time, I was eager to discover what flogging myself would feel like and hoped that it would do me good, rather than having to change my mind and give up my enjoyable habits. So I decided to follow my Master's ritual. It would be such fun to whip myself and experience the joy of pain. I'd never tried it before and had no idea how to begin, but I am an adventurer who is always attracted to weird new experiences. Perhaps beating myself so elegantly would bring me new excitement and I needed the adrenaline. But could that really be the solution to my dilemma? Simply to flog myself, nothing more?

I enthusiastically started to practise the lovely exercise of self-flagellation. During the week I enjoyed my usual pleasurable life more than ever, and then each Sunday before going to church I practised the special healing ritual which my Master had ordered me to do. After an ice-cold shower, I flogged my naked frozen body for one hour until my skin became as bruised and red as a naughty monkey which has disobeyed its owner.

The technique worked well, although the more sore and painful my body became the more sensual I felt and the more I wanted to whip myself. On one hand I was pleasing Heaven, on the other I was increasing my healing power and excitement. I enjoyed the pain, but had to be extremely careful never to allow it under any circumstances to go beyond my limit and take over my whole brain, leaving no room in it for pleasure.

I continued to whip myself vigorously until I became a true master of self-torture. Saints have to learn to tolerate a lot of pain to become healers. I was so happy to have found my answer and longed to teach this beautiful technique of self-purification to others, especially my close friends.

I knew I first had to tell Nunu, a beloved female confidante, how lucky I was to have met a wonderful Master who had rescued me with his whipping method. For two months whilst I was flogging myself I had no contact with her. As soon as we met again, Nunu hugged me tightly and I winced from the pain of my whipped body. She wondered what was going on.

"What's wrong? Did I hurt you?" she asked in surprise.

"My dearest Nunu, I am trembling with happiness and excitement to see you and have great news! I've learned a wonderful new way to empower my healing gift. My life has been completely changed and uplifted. I feel like an angel! I have finally found true salvation."

"You don't look like it!" she replied. "I feel something awful is happening to you. You don't look like the man I used to know. You look so strange, almost as if you're living in another world. I feel you're not being honest with yourself."

"Listen, my dear," I said indignantly, "don't you realise how important my gift is? So many people have told me that my healing comes from God that I have to believe them, because so far I haven't been able to find any other explanation for it. I have to behave as God wishes and flog myself to make Him happy, or He will take his gift back and I'll lose my healing power."

Nunu looked at me with astonishment. "Rached, please don't talk like a masochistic fanatic. It's dreadful to see you acting this way. You are a human being, a good doctor with a loving heart. Why on earth do you have to punish yourself like that?"

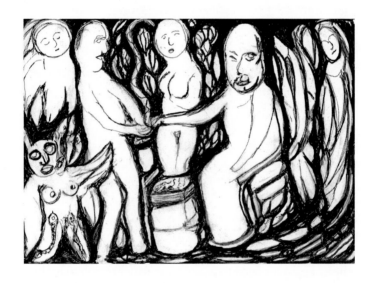

"My dear, please listen and try to understand. I got very confused and discovered that I really understood nothing at all about my healing. I was afraid of losing my gift and needed guidance, so I appealed to a highly regarded Master who knows me well. He convinced me that my only solution was to whip myself."

"Is <u>that</u> what he thought you really needed? Perhaps he was making fun of you and you misinterpreted his words. You are too serious; maybe he had a strange sense of humour which you couldn't understand."

I started to laugh nervously. "Well…" I said "he told me I would enrich my gift by flogging myself with a special whip. I've been following his wisdom by practising his technique since we last met, and now at last I've succeeded. I feel spiritually strong and completely free." Nunu's eyes opened wide. Wagging her finger at me, she drew a deep breath and spoke.

"You don't need a whip - life has already whipped you enough. The whip may be good for a Master, but not for a doctor. You'll kill yourself this way. You must stop at once and live your life like any other normal human being. Your healing comes from your love alone and is itself love. You will only strengthen your healing gift when you live life as it is, following your inner voice guided by love, always with full professional integrity. Do whatever you like or want, as long as it's always done with love. Don't waste time trying to find a rational explanation for the healing process, but accept it for what it is, as long as it serves the well-being of others. First you need to make your patients well; whether you convince them or not by explaining the logic of your work is completely irrelevant."

Thank God! Nunu's wise words brought me the answer I'd been looking for all along. My mind awoke at last from its foggy darkness and I was able to see things clearly again. From now on I'll love myself truthfully and flow with life as it is. I don't need to whip myself in any way! Wherever I go, I'll always listen to my inner voice and nothing else. I'll follow love and do whatever love calls me to.

I became increasingly preoccupied with my medical work. Ever since I had started my practice in Lebanon I had been bombarded with so many patients that there was no time left for any kind of personal life. No time for sleep, no time for a holiday and, worst of all, no time to find a wife with whom to build my future family. And then one day I unexpectedly met a sweet girl; we soon fell in love.

She had polio and walked on sticks, but I loved her so much that my eyes saw only her beauty, not her affliction. Our hearts and minds were intertwined as our love flew with angels and became more than love. More and more, it grew to lift her and free her from paralysis.

She had contracted polio in early childhood. The anterior horn neurons of her spinal cord were invaded by a miserable coxsackie virus. The tiny biological aggressor did its job well, leaving behind its cruel traces. My semi-paralysed sweetheart couldn't blame anybody, only her destiny.

Then one day the Healing Angel came to me in my dreams to inspire me to treat her with healing intimacy. With my hands I stroked all the atrophied muscles of her soft body. Compassion coursed through me, arousing her paralysed feelings and bringing life to her dead spinal cord cells.

We met every day in sessions of God-given intimacy. Shining with all the colours of life, we were two kissing rainbows absorbed in healing light while the soft wind of our love flirted with the golden leaves of autumn. Divine sparks flew from my hands as they pressed upon the deep tissues of my love.

The fire of our passion melted all boundaries. I became a healing artist as my fingers sculpted new life from her atrophied muscles, abandoned in all the past dull years.

Medicine became a song of beauty played by angels on the lyre of Orpheus. The fire of my heart brought back the vital spark to her poor weak flesh. Her thin bones grew full and strong and her dead tissues breathed.

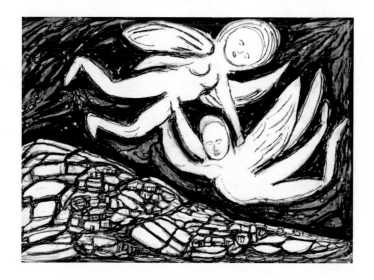

Our heavenly love came to life in the flesh and lifted us above the world. It was divinely sent for her healing, whether we remained together or not. My sweetheart was cured and Raphael descended to embrace us in his joyful dance.

My Wartime Practice

It was 1988 and the Lebanese War had been raging since I first started my practice. Beirut was divided between East and West and armed conflict had become a regular part of our everyday lives.

One day a 31-year-old woman called Lady W visited my Beirut clinic, who had been suffering from migraine for over seven years. She was married to the tough leader of a Lebanese militia group and was the mother of two young children. I studied her case carefully. She was living with her family in a state of extreme anxiety and fear, feeling insecure within herself and in life.

Her husband lived under constant stress. His nature as a leader obliged him to dominate everyone around, even his own family. Lady W was a sensitive woman who suppressed her feelings and needed to protect herself psychologically to avoid conflict. Her migraines were often triggered when her husband asked her to accompany him to parties and other social activities. She got such severe attacks of headache, vomiting fits and hypersensitivity to light that she had to confine herself in a darkened room and take powerful narcotics. It looked as if her migraines were a kind of language through which she was able to refuse her husband's orders.

When I first met Lady W she had a severe headache. I applied a deep healing massage to the spastic muscles of her neck and head and in ten minutes all her pain vanished. I told her that the migraines were caused by physical problems within her body, avoiding any mention of her psychological problem, and explained how the muscular spasms in her neck had put pressure on certain blood vessels connecting to the brain, affecting circulation and causing severe pain.

In my treatment of Lady W I had to take into consideration her upbringing, traditional Lebanese woman's mentality and personal situation. It was impossible under such circumstances for me to try to explain the underlying reasons for her problem, and why in reality she herself was causing the migraines. It would have been out of the question for her to acknowledge that the problem was due to her own mind and her stressful situation. All I could do was to encourage her to become more self-confident and free within in order to tolerate better her difficult life.

Lady W felt very well under the warmth of my healing hands, enjoying their energy and feeling a deep relaxation. Filled with a sense of continuous well-being and no longer vulnerable to anything, she turned into a happy and strong person full of love and inner peace. She became ecstatic, falling in love for the first time with herself as all her spasm and fatigue disappeared. When she left my clinic and arrived home, she met her husband full of cheerful energy. He saw her eyes shining with joy and approached her as usual to absorb her warmth, but felt that his emotional domination over her had lost its power. Unable to get what he was expecting, he became frustrated while his wife stood quietly observing him, full of inner peace and with a new spirit of tolerance for his behaviour.

I started to wonder how her husband might react after my healing. He might become jealous that she had received the good energy and he had not. I imagined him becoming furious and even sending his militia gangsters to kill me on a whim. It is not unusual for things to work like this; it's human nature. It was normal during civil war for people to project hate onto each other and to express it in the language of weapons and killing.

Lady W's husband was a man who had lived a tough life. Maybe he had a severe inferiority complex and had never received real affection or true love. He had probably suffered much abuse in his childhood. If so, my fear was that his jealous emotional state might explode into the murderous language of war. If I were to offer him the same affection I showed his wife could this resolve the dilemma? The time had come to heal. I would have to visit him peacefully and fearlessly to tell him I loved him, imagining that he might have wanted me dead, and had come to ask him to do with me as he pleased. Why not?

Yes, Lady W's husband needed my love! My inner voice called me to see him. I felt genuine compassion for him. He was a beautiful human being but perhaps no-one until now had understood how to relate to him correctly. I went straight to his mansion and called his housekeeper on the intercom to announce that I was the family doctor coming to visit General W The gate opened and I walked in.

The general welcomed me warmly, watching my face and feeling the light of love coming from my eyes as I gazed back at him. He was astonished that I had come to visit him uninvited and was very glad to see me, expressing his gratitude to me for treating and healing his wife. General W politely asked me the reason for my visit and whether he could help me in any way. I replied that I was happy that his wife was cured and had come to visit him without an appointment because I felt his love. He looked into my eyes and felt my sincerity and honesty. He looked like a nice man, not at all as I had seen him in my fantasy. Able to appreciate him perhaps for the first time as a really good person, I wanted our meeting to be harmonious and was very careful not to think badly of him. I started to make small talk.

"How is Madam, your wife?"

"My wife is well. She is now a happy woman. No more migraine or pain. From the day I first met her she was always in pain! Thank you, doctor! You brought the smile back to her face and the happiness to my house. You are really great!"

I became dizzy to hear such sweet words from a man like that and felt that something must have gone badly wrong. Yes! That was it!

The man looked at me through smiling eyes, saying, "Doctor, my wife loves you like an angel sent from God. I am grateful to you for your visit; you must stay here and join us for dinner. My wife is not here. She will return home soon and will be thrilled to see you."

I started to feel myself shaking with fear. Was this man like Stalin, who invited intellectuals to dinner as a reward for their patriotic achievements and then murdered them? After we had finished our meal was he going to shoot me in front of his wife as my reward for having healed her?

Something very weird was going on. Should I make an excuse, refuse his invitation and try to escape? Out of the question: he would feel my fear and kill me immediately. I broke out into a cold sweat and my heart began to pump uncontrollably. I started to hallucinate and saw my body being buried in some dark far-off place.

The general noticed my signs of rising panic and tried to calm me down. Looking sympathetically at me, he started to address me humourously, as if speaking to a child.

"Well, well, doctor! Thank God you decided to come today, otherwise my young friends would have brought you to me dead or alive. I ordered them to bring you here at any price because I missed you. I am pleased to see you and very glad that you are still alive."

There was nothing left for me to do but force myself to smile and surrender. I opened my heart and addressed him with passionate sincerity.

"My dear leader! I come with great love for you. I am yours. Whether you want me dead or alive, I am equally happy. If you want me alive I am your lamb, happy to be slaughtered on the altar of your love."

A beautiful white light shone from his face. He rose from his chair with burning eyes to welcome home his lost angel. His heart became calm at the sight of my sacrifice and tears rolled down his cheeks. Weeping like a child, he took me into his arms exclaiming, "Brother, my dearest brother, I will love you forever. Nobody in the world will ever hurt you. You are the angel of my whole family." Great love burst between us, locking us together. We embraced each other tightly. All boundaries between us collapsed and we were caught up in everlasting friendship.

General W's wife suddenly entered the room. She was astonished to see me in her house and seemed to be very relieved that her husband and I had become such good

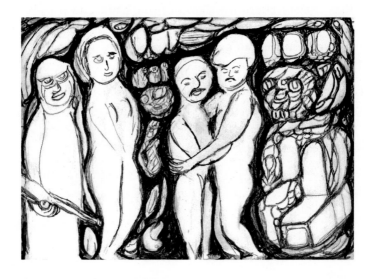

friends. He told her that my visit to him was a great event and ordered her to prepare dinner for us. As she was going to the kitchen, two young men armed with machine guns walked in. They stood to attention in the doorway and told the general that they had spent the whole day trying to find the suspect but with no luck. They didn't know me. Was it me they were looking for? Surely not.

The general chuckled. "The problem is solved!" he said with a laugh. He walked up to them, quickly took away their guns and led them towards me to shake my hand. Realising who I was, they stood flabbergasted and suddenly vanished.

The civil war in Lebanon forced me to become a skilful doctor. It was a real challenge for me to be adaptable and tolerant enough to live under such conditions and to be able to practise medicine. I had to treat many patients who were stressed and traumatised by war. The war in Lebanon was different from any other. It affected people's health with previously unknown symptoms, so I had to discover and invent new ways of treating them.

One hot summer afternoon I was walking home from my Beirut clinic. As I passed by a factory gate I heard sounds of moaning coming from a small guardhouse. Someone was in pain, so I went in and found the janitor lying in agony on the floor and unable to move. I introduced myself and told him I was the right doctor for his case. I saw he was suffering from severe lumbago and confidently told him I could relieve his pain and cure his problem within half an hour. He replied that the factory owner's wife, Lady A., had already gone for an ambulance to take him to hospital. I insisted on treating him anyway in the meantime, and out of desperation he agreed.

I massaged his contracted muscles and he soon felt better. After ten minutes he was free from pain and could stand up to walk. When he saw how quickly his suffering had been relieved, allowing him to move freely, he fell to his knees, kissed the ground and cried with joy.

Lady A soon arrived and was very shocked to see the janitor walking normally, thinking that a miracle had happened. As he danced around merrily, the janitor introduced me and told her what I had done. She looked at me admiringly and was very interested to hear about my work.

Lady A sensed a healing universe working through me and listened enthusiastically to my medical adventures. I explained to her that the essence of my practice consists in adapting orthodox medicine to serve patients more effectively with a unique methodology based on my extensive clinical experience. To help me by making my work better known in society, Lady A invited me to her grand villa to introduce my work to notable representatives of the Lebanese establishment. She enjoyed accompanying me everywhere on my way to help patients. One day we went to visit a friend of hers, Mrs K, a distinguished lady who suffered from a completely paralysed right arm.

At the gate to Mrs K's beautiful mansion stood several heavily armed soldiers. One of them asked us to identify ourselves before we were allowed in. As we entered the drawing room I noticed on the grand piano several photographs of her late husband. He was a brigadier-general in the Lebanese army who had been assassinated at home by terrorists.

Mrs K was thrilled to have me in her house and to hear my healing stories. She sat beside me on the sofa, her eyes shining with the light of compassion, inner strength and wisdom. I felt how charismatic and special a lady she was. She showed me her paralysed right hand and started to tell me her story.

"Last year, as my husband and I lay asleep at two o'clock in the morning, several gunmen burst into our bedroom and fired dozens of bullets into us from silenced machineguns. My husband was hit by twenty-eight bullets and died immediately, while I was seriously wounded with nineteen bullets in my body. One of our neighbours sensed trouble and rushed in to find us bathed in pools of blood. I had already lost consciousness. He quickly called an ambulance to take us to the hospital's emergency ward. The nurses who examined us found that we had no pulse and no detectable heartbeat. They thought that we were both dead and put us in the refrigerator until the following day. The army leadership planned to bury us in an official national ceremony. Next morning the undertakers came to remove our corpses and prepare them for burial. They put my husband's body into his coffin, but when they started to pick me up one of them thought he could feel a tiny pulse and immediately called the resident doctor to examine me. The doctor was amazed to find signs of life in me. They took me into intensive care and sent my husband to his grave. I had twenty-five operations, one of which took twelve hours. The surgeons extracted fifteen bullets from my body and I still have several left in me which they couldn't remove. As you can see, I'm still alive but my right arm is useless!"

I asked her to describe what kind of injuries had caused her paralysis.

"The brachial plexus was burnt by gunfire. A bullet severed my median nerve and several bones in my hand were shattered. The neurosurgeon suggested a nerve transplant but we decided it was pointless."

The lady was wise, shrewd and pious. She was a heroine who had conquered death. Her bitter experience had produced in her an indomitable spirit. I was convinced that such a strong character would respond extremely positively to my

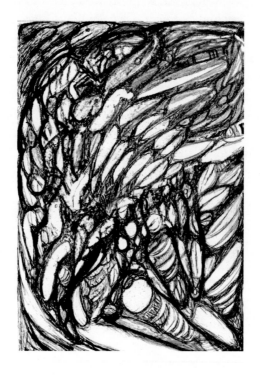

treatment. I started to work with her in my own way, and after ten minutes her paralysed fingers started to move. It is unheard of for muscles to regain their function when their nerves are severed – but it happened.

After a month of further treatment, Mrs K visited her neurosurgeon to show him her perfectly functioning arm.

After a thorough examination, he was utterly bewildered and baffled. What had happened defied all known medical possibilities. The story of how I had healed her hand became famous, and further inspired me to look for new methods of treating paralysis, exploring ways of stimulating neural centres with new programmes to rewire neurons and induce healing feedback.

Later on, I studied a number of my recovered cases similar to that of Lady K Surprisingly, the medical tests for a few of them showed that even though their nerves were still severed their arms were working perfectly.

Turning Point

Early one morning in January 1990 an insane war suddenly exploded in East Beirut. Two Lebanese military groups had started heavy fighting with each other. One army was occupying the district of Jdeidet el Metn, turning the Etihad Gallery by my home into the battle front line, while the other army had established their fighting front at the Gallery Khabbaz next to my clinic in Sad el Bauchrieh. The main line of fire between them was along Boulevard Sin el Fil leading from my apartment to my clinic. These two military groups were furiously bombarding each other with rockets and shells. The sky was ripped apart by the continuous thunder of cannon and heavy machine gun fire.

A rocket invaded my apartment while I was lying on my bed. The kitchen exploded and everything was thrown upside down. My bed fell on top of me, saving me from shrapnel. I jumped up in panic, looking to see if I was still in one piece. Suffocated by smoke and dust I reeled out, dragging my body from the ruins looking for an escape. Had the stairs of the building fallen down? I looked through my third-floor window, wondering whether I should jump out from it before the whole building collapsed under the heavy shelling.

I saw another building on fire at the end of the boulevard. My clinic was ablaze, darkening the sky with heavy smoke.

It was being bombarded by cannon shells sent from beside my home.

I fled from my apartment and rushed downstairs as several more rockets smashed into it and ran into the street in my pyjamas. A tank battle was raging about me. Snipers were shooting from everywhere. Bullets and bombs rained death along the way as I ran across the road with many others towards the nearest underground shelter.

Almost a hundred of us stayed huddled together for ten days with no food in that shelter. We were all trapped down there by a war that could have buried us alive at any moment. Above us, a storm of shooting, killing and devastation moved from street to street.

With every strong vibration from the explosions that frequently shook the walls of the shelter like an earthquake, our breath stopped and cold sweat covered our bodies. Our throats were choked by the smell of gunpowder and charred bodies beneath the ruins. We groped through the dark in terror and slept with rats and cockroaches on the cold damp ground. The underground cavern was our burial crypt. We crept through its gloom, searching for any tiny scrap of hope that might keep us alive.

Everyone was moaning in fear and grief. Everyone had his own way of facing death. Our hearts were wounded by cries of pain coming from every corner. The deafening sound of gunfire and explosions had paralysed our minds.

A rocket fell outside; it exploded and everything burst into flames. Four more rockets hit the building above us. One of them penetrated three floors and blew up. A piece of the ceiling fell onto a woman's foot and broke it. She fell screaming to the floor. A man lying against the wall was shaken by the force of the explosion and his whole body went into spasm, his shoulders frozen, his back twisted, his legs rigid. He collapsed, racked with pain. Two women were smashed together by the blast and fell traumatised. A woman behind me was vomiting from severe migraine. An old man was dying of asthma, suffocated by the fumes from outside. A young woman was so shocked that her blood pressure rocketed and she collapsed with a stroke. Others lay on the damp floor as pale as corpses. They were starving and life was fading. For ten days there was no way of getting any food. Mothers and children were crying from hunger. A woman in the sixth month of pregnancy was in agony and about to lose her child.

In a corner of the shelter a young couple sat in a passionate embrace. They were as absorbed in each other as if there had been no war. Another couple smiled at each other, their happiness shining through the clouds of sadness. They had fallen in love and were delighted to be trapped there together.

We all shared our pain and suffering in that shelter. We were looking desperately for hope to come from somewhere. But who would bring it? Who would come to rescue us?

I lost my clinic. I lost my home. I lost my kingdom. I was buried alive in the shelter. I couldn't stand to see how war was killing my people, how my loved ones were about to die. I am a doctor, a human being, a sufferer.

No, no, no! Enough tragedy. I will never allow war to crush our spirit. War had stolen all I had but would never steal my soul or destroy my love. I will never surrender. War

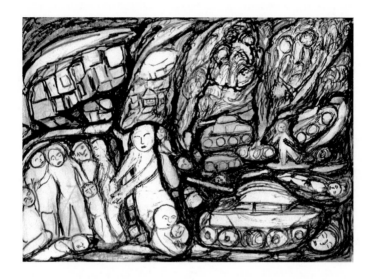

may destroy clinics, hospitals, pharmacies and medical equipment, but never the human fire in our souls.

Suddenly a great universal compassion took me over. I saw myself living beyond space and time, becoming a temple of healing, my hands turning into tools for healing. My old doctor and clinic vanished and my real clinic appeared within. I felt a new power rising in me, stronger than the volcano of war, coming to wipe away all pain in the shelter.

The woman with the broken foot stood before me, crying, "Doctor, Doctor, help me, help me!" Blood was pouring from her wound and nothing could stop it. As soon as I touched her I saw the bleeding cease and her injuries disappear. As I turned towards the young woman with the stroke, I saw her already recovering. A whirling light filled the shelter while my arms were reaching out to help and instantly everyone's affliction was healed.

The fog of sadness was blown away and the light of joy rose up to shine in our souls. Great peace came to wipe away the hell of war. A soft, warm zephyr flowed through us, quietening the din as silence descended.

All of a sudden the racket of gunfire and explosions started to abate. Only a few gunshots broke the silence now and then. I left the shelter and started to live and heal in the midst of war as if it no longer existed. I was guided by a great compassion that turned suffering into joy and war into illusion. I no longer needed a clinic or a home and surrendered to the healing will, freely guiding me wherever I went.

For six months amidst the war in Lebanon I travelled from shelter to shelter and from home to home with only my empty hands. I was welcomed everywhere to eat, sleep and heal.

I continued to live in Beirut, spending every night in damp, dark shelters to the sound of intense shelling. Under the showers of rockets which were devastating buildings and killing people, I went everywhere to help my patients.

My mind was above the war and didn't realise the extreme danger threatening me from all sides. I was completely absorbed by thoughts of how to heal those who were suffering. A bomb, a bullet or even a tiny piece of shrapnel could have killed me at any time. My friend Emil, the Lebanese Ambassador to Bucharest, wanted to rescue me from the danger of Beirut's random bombing so he invited me to stay with him in Romania. With no other alternative I accepted.

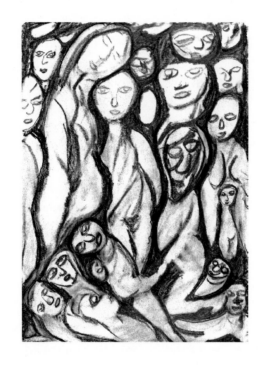

Healing Journey

One day as I was relaxing by the pool of the Diplomatic Club in Bucharest enjoying the sunlight and cool water a beautiful young girl came up to sit near me. She glanced sideways at me with an innocent warmth as her golden hair fluttered across her shining eyes. I was very attracted to her and wanted to get closer. She wished to talk to me and not talk to me, to come near and to move away. How could I best charm her?

Watching her in the late September sun, I noticed that there was something odd about her right hand and leg. She rose and walked with chaotic, swaying steps to the end of the pool. It looked as if she was trying to conceal some weakness and didn't want me to see any flaw in her gorgeous body.

I was curious to know what her problem was. It seemed likely that she had suffered a head injury at birth and that the compression of the forceps had resulted in a partial paralysis of her right side.

I was moved to get up and walk towards the girl. "She is lovely, you can help her. Go and touch such beauty with your healing hands," my heart whispered to me. The girl with the golden hair saw that I wanted to talk to her and walked back towards me.

"My dear sir, you are looking at me as if you know me. Have we met before?"

"Allow me to introduce myself to you. I am Dr Rached Daoud from Lebanon and I'm staying here as the guest of our ambassador. I noticed how you were walking and see you have a problem with your hand and leg. I can tell you honestly, I have a solution for it and would love to help you. Give me your hand and let me treat it with my special massage. I'm sure that in a few minutes you'll notice the difference and will be able to move your fingers properly for the first time in your life."

"Thank you for offering me your help," she replied. "I'm comfortable with the way I am and will be happy just to talk with you." She took a chair and sat down beside me.

"My name is Natalia. I am the daughter of a Yugoslavian diplomat. I am very happy to meet you."

Looking at her sweet baby face, I took her right hand and held it gently. She smiled and said, "What soft warm hands you have." While we went on talking I started to massage her hand. She enjoyed it and allowed me do my work. In a little while, and for the first time in her life, her fingers started to move.

As she felt her paralysed hand come back to life, a smile lit up her face and her blue eyes glistened. She cried out, "Oh my God! I can move my fingers! I can use my hand. I can't believe it. Now I can do so many things I couldn't do before!"

All the diplomats sitting around the pool heard the commotion and looked towards us to see what was happening. They thought a miracle must have occurred and gathered round so I could treat them too. Everyone was overjoyed at what had just happened and started to celebrate in a spontaneous party.

News of this episode spread quickly within the ambassadorial community and I soon found myself being invited to treat other diplomats.

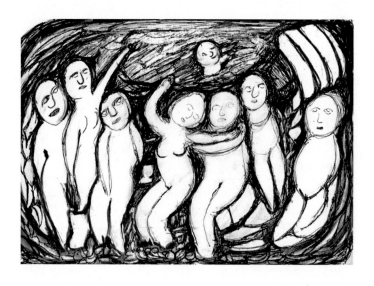

After staying for three months with my friend Emil, I became tired of diplomatic social life with its endless parties and wanted to escape Bucharest. But to where? Romania is such a beautiful country, with its gorgeous Carpathian Mountains, shining lakes and green valleys. Why not go to Cluj-Napoca, the beautiful old city where I had studied medicine for seven years?

Cluj, where I lived as a medical student, is my favourite place in the world. I grew up there, not only as a physician but also as a poet. She nourished me with her deeply-rooted European spirituality and raised me with her charming old Austro-Hungarian culture, enriching and warming my soul with so much love and attracting me with her romantic life.

So I took the next express train to Cluj late that evening and as soon as I arrived there next morning I went for a stroll through its ancient streets and alleyways, revisiting its cafés and restaurants. I found myself once again enjoying the exciting bohemian life of my student days. How lovely it would be to bump into some of my old friends and maybe meet new ones, too. Perhaps some of them had read my books; it would be wonderful to gather together, enjoying poetry like we used to in the old days.

As I meandered through the ancient cobbled streets of the town centre I suddenly spied my old friends Badica and Ovidiu sitting in Croco, our old student café. We were overjoyed to meet again for the first time in six years. I was thrilled to hear how well they had been doing after the fall of the Communist regime. They were equally interested to find out what I'd been up to since last we met and how I'd been able to survive the Lebanese war.

When my friends saw my delight in being with them again and felt my great love for Cluj, they were filled with enthusiasm to create and share new cultural events, as we did in our idyllic student days. They suggested inviting our friends and anyone else who might be interested in coming to a recital of my poetry, so we agreed to have our cultural event in the hall of the Medical Institute. It was an excellent idea to recite my poetry where I'd studied medicine and I didn't want to miss such an opportunity.

But I had none of my books with me and could remember only a few poems. I needed more. But how? I simply had to invent some quickly. Maybe before the meeting a few glasses of palinca, the famously strong prune vodka of the region, would answer my question. It would provide courage and confidence, and I was quite sure it would inspire me to compose spontaneous poetry for my audience.

Drinking the palinca about ten minutes before entering the hall would be perfect. I would feel splendid and in that euphoric state magnificent poetry easily enters my head. It would be marvellous when the palinca brought its poetic spirit to me, and if not it wouldn't make any difference. Alcohol would take the blame for any poetic failure, not me, and my friends would simply be pleased to see me drunk and happy. In the best old Romanian tradition, an inebriated gentleman is always forgiven for any misbehaviour and whatever he does is seen as amusing.

So, like a generous peasant trying to boost his confidence, I quickly drank half a bottle of the best palinca. Feeling greatly improved, I strode into the hall where a huge crowd was eagerly awaiting my entrance. As they started to cheer and applaud me I felt very thrilled and proud of myself. I started to address my audience with improvised verse expressing compassion, but my mind had betrayed me - it was so blank that I couldn't even remember my name.

The atmosphere in the hall was very strange; something was distorting the reality of space and time. Shapes started to change form. Everything in the room was vibrating and looked as if it was about to fly away. I tried to say something but no poetry came from my mouth, only blabber. What happened to my brain, for God's sake? Where had all my poetry gone? Who could possibly have stolen it? Looking around to find out what might be happening, I saw only floating shadows. Was my poetic Muse hiding behind them? I stretched out my hands to reach Her and my fingers grasped thin air. Where was my Muse? Why had she betrayed me? Poetic angel, come at once to save me! Reaching out my hands further and further to touch something, even if only one single hair of my goddess, I staggered and my shaking hands fell instead onto the head of a passing ten-year-old girl and grabbed both her ears. What am I doing? What is happening? My hands and face were burning and the girl burst into tears, screaming, "Mother, mother!"

My God - what had I done to the poor girl? Had I torn her ears off?

The entire audience fell to their knees, shouting wordlessly and frantically gesticulating.

Oh! Oh! What's happening? I looked around in terror. Did they want to kill me for hurting the poor girl? I saw myself being torn to pieces by the mob.

But no...with mouths agape, their faces shone with the light of awe and love, not hate...

Suddenly, I heard a voice calling out from their midst uttering one sentence: "Laura, Laura, you are speaking and hearing, you are healed!"

The voice from the crowd wasn't angry with me. It had nothing against me. It looked as if it was going to spare my life after all. Relief flooded through me.

Whose voice was speaking? What was it? Who is Laura? Someone here seems to have been healed but surely it had nothing to do with me. I only came here to recite poetry and have fun.

But still…something very mysterious was going on…

As I peered into the surrounding shadows they became fainter. Aha! The fog began to lift and I started to see things more clearly. Had I heard right? Had someone called Laura really been healed? Where was she?

"Who is Laura?" I shouted. The little girl rushed up to me with her mother and hugged me. Her mother seized my hand and kissed it tearfully, saying, "This is the holy hand which healed my deaf-mute daughter Laura as she passed by."

Something very strange must have provoked a healing explosion. But surely not me? It couldn't have been because of me…then who or what? I still felt blank and woozy. What on earth was holy about a funny fool who could hardly stand up straight or even remember his name? Can the shaky hands of a drunkard heal anybody?

Suddenly an old woman appeared by my side and started tugging at my sleeve. She was babbling and jabbering at me. What on earth could she possibly have wanted? She was hideous, grimacing at me through smiling broken teeth. She pointed to her damaged left eye, which was full of pus and blood. What made her think I was interested in it? Why was she showing me something so disgusting? I hadn't come to see such disturbing things. I was in Cluj to enjoy poetry and pleasure, nothing else.

Did she want me to heal her? Whatever could have given her such an idea? Who might have told her? Had she heard what Laura's mother said about me, that I had healed her daughter? How could she believe such nonsense! I looked around and made a last attempt to find my Muse and recite my beautiful poetry.

More light was coming into the room and the faces of the people were now a bit clearer. I noticed some of my doctor friends there. One of them, Ioan, my best friend at medical school, came up to me with Laura and shook my hand. Introducing her as his patient, he told me that something really strange had just happened to her in the hall. As soon as my hands had touched her ears, she could hear voices for the first time in her life.

Ioan took me by the shoulder, introduced me to the half-blind woman and explained that she was his mother. He had told her a lot about me. I asked him what she was asking me for so insistently and with a soft laugh he replied that his mother already knew whom I was. She just needed my attention and all I had to do to satisfy her was simply to lay my hands onto her infected eye for a few moments, exactly as I had done with Laura's ears. Ioan's mother smiled sweetly at me - all of a sudden she was starting to look beautiful.

I didn't take Ioan too seriously. I knew his love of fantasy but, out of respect for his mother and as a psychological prop, I agreed to go along with his unlikely plan for me to touch her damaged eye. I did as my dear colleague suggested and after a few minutes I removed my hands from her eye. As soon I had done so she started to shriek, "Oh my God! I can see! Light has entered my eye!"

Her yells shook the whole building of the Institute of Medicine and collapsed my rational medical mind. Examining the old woman's left eye, I saw that her cornea and iris had become clear and regained their natural colour. Neither spots of blood nor signs of pus could be seen any more.

I was utterly terrified by this bizarre phenomenon. My medically-conditioned mind drove me to escape from this healing nightmare and deny its truth, but I felt paralysed by the conflict of opposites. Falling to my knees with my forehead on the woman's feet, I raised my hands in supplication, crying, "Thank you! Thank you! Your presence here has brought me to God! Thank you! You have healed me of scepticism."

And of scepticism I <u>was</u> healed.

The great assembly saw in me a knight struck down from his horse by the sword of light. I became unfathomable.

A hubbub of confusion broke through the silent atmosphere of the room.

"With whom is he speaking?"…"Is he speaking to God?"… "Is he mad?"…"Is he completely unaware that he has just healed her?"…"If he didn't, then who or what did heal that old woman?"

The answer to all these questions was silence. Into this charged atmosphere a gypsy beggar came through the doors supporting his body on crutches. The sound of their loud tapping broke the stillness. Perhaps he had smelt the fire of healing coming from the building or was prompted to enter by an inner voice. He extended his hands, not for money but to ask me to heal his legs, paralysed by polio.

He was tired of begging for so many years and wanted to walk and work. The disabled man threw himself at my feet and begged me to help him. People started to whisper, "Who told this young gypsy to come here? How did he get in here?"

I felt unable to do anything for him but my hands were guided to press on the weak paralysed muscles of his limbs. It seemed as if he saw himself fully cured and that his faith exceeded mine. Feeling grateful and stretching himself with the confidence of his piety, he rose to leave the room and walked out with tears twinkling in his eyes, dragging his legs and leaving his crutches behind.

Professor Hauescu, a rheumatologist who had once taught me medicine, was watching me in disbelief. He limped up to me suspiciously and spoke in a hoarse, shaking voice, addressing me as if I was still his student.

"Colleague, are you such a doer of miracles?...if you have really cured that gypsy beggar...we were good friends and you were my best student...I'm sure you can also cure my hemiplegia!"

I examined him. His right arm and leg presented a slight muscular weakness due to an old stroke. I had successfully treated many such cases and then simply left the patient to do exercise, so I was delighted that Professor Hauescu had offered me a golden opportunity to demonstrate my healing power to everybody.

"Colleague, I can most assuredly help you," I declared, puffing out my chest with professional pride. "You will be pleasantly surprised to learn in only a few moments that your leg will be better than new. Let us begin! I will now demonstrate to you how easily I can release the spasm in your right leg with my unique advanced physiotherapeutic rehabilitation manoeuvres which will restore your normal muscular synergism by perfectly coordinating your antagonistic extensor-flexor functions."

"Colleague, what you are saying is completely and perfectly logical," replied Hauescu with a weak smile. "It all sounds extremely scientific. Here is my leg, here is my hand. Cure them! I want to see how my best student has progressed."

My chest burst with even more pride to have been chosen by such a high medical authority to demonstrate my brilliance. I listened to the inner voice on which I had always depended, telling me that I would now prove that I was the greatest doctor in the world and had a golden opportunity to demonstrate it to someone with whom I shared a special medical language.

I expertly positioned my hands to manipulate his muscles and demonstrate my magical curing ability, but soon noticed that his case was proving to be more difficult than I had anticipated. Unfortunately, it was also beginning to appear as if it might in fact turn out to be totally impossible. Sweating with exhaustion and completely drained of all energy after thirty minutes of futile effort, I realised that my hard work had all been in vain.

Bloody hell! Where had my healing energy gone? I was shocked and depressed at the lack of results and felt wretched, worse than a stray dog. How could I have succeeded with the paralysed Romanian gypsy but not with my professor's tiny muscular weakness? I wanted to be a hero to such an exalted personage, not to a poor beaten-down beggar. It was really unfair!

The professor, looking at me with ill-concealed contempt, delivered his final judgement.

"You, who were my best student! I have tested your ambitious claims and have found them to be completely false. You said that you could cure my leg but obviously can't, as your medical colleagues will all have witnessed. I regret to have to inform you that you have lost your way and appear to be a medical inadequate. I am bitterly disappointed by your failure to fulfil the high hopes I had placed in you. I advise you to stop playing your silly games at once. Either go home or start to recite some poetry!"

He left the room in a huff with most of my ex-colleagues, leaving a handful of stoical physicians who chose to remain by my side. Frustrated by what had happened and fed up with my need to prove myself to others, I was really upset by Hauescu's imperious attack on me. Why had he behaved like that? Did he imagine that I was still his student and had to pass his examination? Why had I let him treat me like a fumbling schoolboy?

Forget about him. Forget about myself. Returning to my audience, I opened my heart with love and warmth. Everyone in the room had lost interest in my curing their physical infirmities. No-one wanted to see their hero fall for a second time.

The room became filled with compassion as healing started to work in another dimension, treating the wounds of the heart and removing the darkness of the mind. I saw myself sitting in the shadow of the unknown and felt my spirit living through past millennia, shaded by the ancient Civilisation of Love, listening to the voice of silence...

And Silence spoke. *I have come from the land which once gave light to the world, from caves protecting the spark of love, to listen with you to the divine cry of your hearts before they were strangled by Mammon. Free yourself by the light that comes only from above and not from below! With my words receive the torch to guide you through the vastness of the great Universe of Love.*

Mystical delirium suddenly filled the minds and flooded the hearts of the crowd, which had lost all awareness of time and space. Everyone was staring at me with burning intensity, as if I was their saviour. Their superstitious hunger awoke me from my trance and filled me with rage. Angrily I bellowed, "I am not what you think I am. I am only a miserable helpless human being like the rest of you. Nobody forced me to come here. It just happened and I'm enjoying it. We're all here together to have fun and for me to embrace your love."

By now the audience was completely convinced that I was their Awaited One.

I became upset by the way they wanted to turn me into their guru and had no wish to lead them up the garden path, wanting them to live their reality and learn to have faith in themselves without being blinded by emotional addiction. Without condemning them, I can understand how it's often more comfortable for us to stay stuck in our habits without working on ourselves. I always encourage individuals to govern themselves responsibly rather than being slaves to any idea or image. Our thoughts should be realistic and our minds remain free and unconditioned.

Wishing to help everyone to see me more objectively, I detached myself completely from the emotional maelstrom rushing through Cluj and rose to address the multitude from my enlightened viewpoint. In a voice filled with compassion, I called on them to manifest their inner truth.

Two charming young girls were so moved emotionally by my energy that they wanted to come and hug me. I stupidly shouted at them, "I warn you, don't come near me thinking I'm some kind of saint! Don't trust me with your bodies and throw yourselves into my lap. I am a wicked human being and my obscene nature can easily burst out."

Nothing I could say or do seemed to deter anyone from looking up to me as a superior being. I had at all costs to clean out this paranoid image from their minds and replace it with a shared devotion to the high principles of human love through which we had originally intended to meet. Seeing before me several bottles of palinca, I started to drink like a madman and behave like a drunken Romanian peasant.

As the alcohol did its work, it started to influence my balance and I collapsed to the floor, my shoulder smashing into someone's foot with the full force of my body behind it. There was a terrible cracking sound and I heard a man scream as he jumped up in furious pain. I knew with sickening certainty that I had broken all the bones of his foot and gave up in complete defeat. Nothing mattered any more. Regardless of how many more broken bones or torn ears for which I might be blamed, I knew I was completely done for.

Suddenly I saw the man laughing and embracing me. Had his great pain driven him mad? I raised my hands protectively to cover my throat and face as I waited for his blows to rain down on me.

Wrong again! Everyone was by now laughing hysterically. I beheld a woman pouring more palinca into a glass and holding it out to me. "Drink more, Master. This prune spirit is holy! Drink, drink! Fill yourself with its healing power!" "I got it, I got it!" I muttered to myself.

In my drunken stupor I had accidentally fallen on a man's calcified foot. The impact had freed his frozen joints, causing the cracking sound and curing him. As is the custom in Romania, people assumed that the palinca had inspired me to perform yet another healing miracle, and out of their natural kindness they wanted to make me even more drunk.

I was again struck speechless by the weirdness of my situation. Then, from the gloom, there appeared a radiance scattering the mist of my mind and breaking open the gates of my heart. What could it be? It shone like an angel from paradise, landing deep within me to calm my gale and guide my ragged sails to a safe haven. Was it my long-sought poetic Muse?

Surely not. Perhaps she was my love muse, a goddess sent for my thirsty heart, for whom I had originally come. I was struck by the sight of her, a beautiful young woman offering her hands to lift me from the floor and embracing me, like an angel opening up her wings to carry me aloft above all wretchedness. Surely she <u>was</u> my healing poetic muse! My goddess of beauty! Her sweet looks inflamed my soul with ecstasy, filling me with love energy.

She was Florfina, the princess of my heart, by whom I was guided to Cluj. From the first, she had been following me in the audience with her radiant eyes drunk with beauty. She was there for my salvation, to rescue me from the emotional delirium and chaos flooding through Cluj!

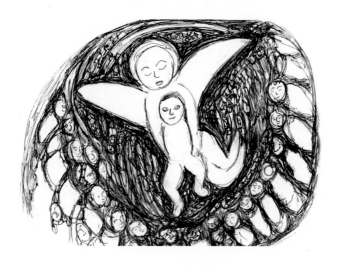

Turning me into a child, the angelic Florfina took my hands and flew with me high above everything towards the world of peace, somewhere where no-one would follow us.

I had to leave Romania before the emotionally unstable Balkan spirit drove me crazy. I needed to go somewhere else, hopefully to a country with more stability and discipline, where the climate would help me to develop further my practice with compatible professionals.

I was lucky enough to be invited to London by a top medical authority, a psychiatrist and alternative medicine researcher. He was impressed by my achievements as a doctor of the impossible, and had a particular interest in paranormal studies and the phenomenology of delusion. He introduced himself as a famous and highly respected world scientist interested in the study of inexplicable healing phenomena. Through his charm and imagination, he had been able to play with psychoanalytical concepts in an attempt to invent a model for a postmodernist shamanic alchemy. He was looking hard for a new kind of dark energy within the mind to justify and explain his quasi-scientific theories of healing.

I was fascinated to meet anyone who might be able to offer a rational, scientific and objective basis for hitherto inexplicable healing processes. Only then will it become possible to build a healing educational system for the future advancement of medicine.

As I entered Dr X's elegant Hampstead mansion, I found myself confronted by a most charismatic person. Gazing at me quizzically with his dark penetrating eyes, he impressed me with his appearance, a look much to my taste. I felt that we had a lot in common and shared similar intellectual likes and dislikes. He had the powerful beard of Sigmund Freud, the charming expression of Carl Jung and the wild hair of Albert Einstein. Pointing his finger towards the ceiling like Ferdinand de Lesseps opening the Suez Canal, in order to indicate that healing is a process by which we connect ourselves to our higher awareness, he explained to me his whole mind-body-spirit model and how he taught it to doctors. As I started to enumerate to Dr X my own accomplishments, using conventional medical terminology, he interrupted me to say that my work was based on a natural healing gift from Higher Intelligence and that I was a medium who had to become fully attuned with It to accomplish my purpose. I agreed with him, or at

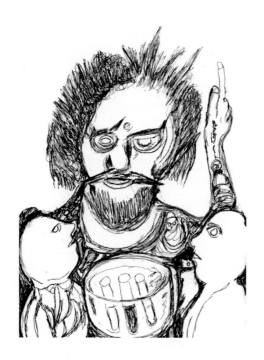

least with his good intentions, and asked him as a doctor to suggest a professional description for my practice.

"You are a healer. You therefore practise healing energy medicine," he replied.

"What's that?"

"Through your hands you channel the energy that heals."

"What kind of energy, and how can I detect, control and use it?"

"It is a healing cosmic energy. As a part of the universe you're fully connected to it. Universal consciousness transmits its information and energy through you to heal others. You are simply its channel, a chosen person sent to heal the sick. The world needs your healing energy!"

"How can I prove that when I apply my hands to my patients there is energy flowing through them, and what kind of energy it is?"

"The answer is obvious! Just look at the fantastic healing results you bring to your patients. From my point of view as a highly qualified professional scientist, the only possible explanation for it is Energy."

"Dr X, how can I measure, control and exploit this healing cosmic energy? Is there any research facility in which to do this? One day I'd like to see a paper written about it. Maybe my hands could even produce enough energy to make special healing batteries to recharge my patients. Why not, sir? I'm very happy to hear it from an authority like you.

"Science recognises four fundamental potential energies, electric, magnetic, strong and weak nuclear, and knows how to use them through technology to produce power. It would be great if we could add my energy to the list. Then, sir, I would be number five...maybe my fifth energy is a free one, even more important than gravity and dark matter!"

"Please do not complicate things." Dr X removed his glasses, scratched his beard and peered at me. "Please don't interpret me literally or mechanistically. Listen carefully to my concepts and understand I'm only trying to help you. Why are you so obsessed, as if you were trying to invent a new atom bomb? Just accept things as they are. All I know is that you are full of bio-energy and must go on using it to help others."

"Sorry for being so pragmatic and obsessed with physics," I replied. "I think you are using the term 'energy' poetically and not scientifically, as a metaphor to describe healing. Anyway, your energy concept has nothing to do with my work. Can you define what I do in another way more appropriate for me and more convincing to others?"

"OK, just call your work spiritual healing and tell people you are a spiritual healer."

"That's the wrong term to describe my work. It's used for healing within a religious establishment. Spiritual healing outside religious establishments could sometimes be misinterpreted."

"Then just call yourself a healer with a God-sent gift."

"If my healing comes from God I'm going to need written proof from Him, or no one will believe it! Can you get it for me?"

"Why don't you go and ask Him for it?" he replied, and we both laughed. His wife came in from the kitchen with a pot of tea, interrupting us to say that we shouldn't talk so much about ourselves and needed to keep quiet about our work. I agreed with her that I had to learn how to heal others quietly without trying to explain anything. She was happy to hear it and asked me to fix her frozen shoulder, which I did further comment.

Dr X subsequently suggested that I would benefit from meeting several medical practitioners who might possibly be interested in my work. One of them was Cordelia, who invited me to the hospital where she practised as a surgeon. She claimed to be a spiritual healer, specialising in distant healing assisted by several volunteer energy workers.

As I entered her office I immediately felt her authority. "What do you think you're doing here?" she demanded impatiently.

"I have come for the advancement of medicine and to collaborate with my British colleagues," I firmly replied. "I am here to introduce to them my unique, new and revolutionary medical discoveries, which have proved successful in many cases previously considered incurable." Dr Cordelia looked at me in disbelief, as if I was a snobbish oriental braggart.

"Now look here, young man! You're in England and had better learn to shut up and listen. You were directed here so that our country can heal you from your Middle Eastern negativity. I'm going to send you to my spiritual master John for help. He is my guide through whom I communicate with my daughter, who died ten years ago."

So I went to meet John, curious to learn more. My train arrived in time for tea at his pretty cottage in the Surrey countryside. He welcomed me from the kitchen table, where he sat with his plump girlfriend Arabella, a renowned karmic regression clairvoyant. Before I even had time to introduce myself, Arabella pointed her finger at me and declared, "Hello! We've met before, you know. We were together in a past life on the island of Atlantis in the year 10001 BC. John, do you remember?"

"Oh yes, of course I do!" replied John, smiling faintly.

"How could I ever forget him? I can also clearly remember our arduous journey to Bethlehem, where we were all present at the birth of Master Jesus." He handed me a mug of warm tea.

Looking searchingly at me, he continued. "So, you see, we've known each other for more than twelve thousand years! What extraordinary lives we have all shared together across the vastness of time. You are my best and oldest friend! We have been together since the beginning of civilisation." I looked at these two people stunned, uncertain whether I had heard correctly, and took a sip of tea.

John led me to the living room and sat me down in a comfortable leather armchair so that he could open up my psyche and cleanse me, as Cordelia had insisted.

"Sit! Sit down!" he commanded. I sank deeply into his armchair.

"Close, close your eyes!" I shut my eyes.

"What do you see now that your eyes are closed?"

"I see nothing, John."

"Open your eyes wide! Now close them again and tell me exactly what you see." I gave no reply.

"What do you see?" John kept saying.

He went on asking me the same question again and again until at last I came up with the right answer. "Now I see an angel, John! It's absolutely amazing! I can really see an angel!" It was exactly what he wanted to hear.

"Excellent!" he crowed. "Open your eyes and look at the wall. The angel is watching you from there. You are now the servant of Light. Witness before you the angel who helped Christ, whom I have just revealed to you. Together we shall heal the British Isles - it is for this that you have been incarnated!

"Go, return to your home. You have received a great message and now clearly understand your mission. You have to leave right away, as I have to go upstairs to receive my daily message from my spiritual guide, Master Clonthroxides of the Andromeda galaxy. I am his Chosen Vessel."

I left John's cottage feeling dizzy and bemused, really happy to have escaped from him. Arriving back in London, I took a taxi from Victoria Station to Notting Hill, but asked the driver to drop me off in Hyde Park because I didn't have enough cash to pay for the whole trip. As he reached out towards me to take his money he winced and cried out in pain. He had twisted his back.

I have never been able to see someone in pain and remain indifferent. His back trouble would make it difficult for him to drive his taxi and he might suffer financial loss. I knew I could cure him easily in five minutes and implored him to let me help. At first he was suspicious, but I persuaded him to allow me to try. I made him wrap his arms around a tree trunk so I could get to work on his back. Within three minutes I had relaxed his contracted muscles and he was cured. He thought it was a miracle.

"Amazing! Amazing!" he exclaimed. "How on earth did you do that? You just touched me and I was instantly cured. I've never seen anything like it before. It's a bloody miracle! Only Jesus Christ heals like that!"

"I never perform miracles," I answered, "I'm just a good doctor." The driver stretched his back in disbelief and looked at me admiringly. "Where are you from?" he asked.

"I'm from Lebanon. Have you heard of it?"

"Of course I have! Lebanon is the Holy Land where Our Lord performed many miracles and healed the Canaanite woman - oh my God!! I saw in a spiritual book that Christ will appear this year in England. He'll come here from Asia and Lebanon's in Asia! He'll heal everybody in Britain from all its negativity...it's bloody amazing! You are our Messiah!"

I shrugged. "OK, if you say so. I'm really just a physician here to help sufferers." From then on he refused to leave me and reverently volunteered to be my guide for the rest of the day. Along the way, he couldn't stop babbling about how blessed he was to have discovered me, the awaited Messiah.

"My Lord, I am Bill. You have come to us in England to heal the possessed and cast out our demons. Master, please let me take you to my home - I need you to cast out the horrible demon haunting my wife."

Bill really needed my help and I listened to him with pity. He was a good-hearted simple London Cockney who had willingly provided me with his amusing company, so I accepted his request to heal his wife. Perhaps she was simply suffering from depression.

We arrived in the late afternoon at Bill's ground floor flat in North London. His young wife was lying on the sofa eating chocolates, her eyes full of wicked Irish charm.

"Hello, love!" Bill greeted her. "Have you had a good day? Look who I've brought home! I met him this morning in my taxi at Victoria Station, and when I dropped him off at Hyde Park I hurt my back again. I was in terrible pain but he fixed it. He performed a miracle! He's the Messiah we were talking about! Remember the prophecies I heard saying he'll come to England this year and many will know Him by his healing? That's exactly what has just happened to me! He's here to bless our flat and heal you - aren't we lucky to have Him here!"

His wife gestured to a nearby chair and I sat down. Bill nodded his approval and left us alone together. As soon as he was out of the room, she laughed and wagged her finger at her head. I started to introduce myself.

"I am a great and famous physician from Lebanon. I have cured your husband's back immediately simply by my touch and I am now here to see you."

"Oh, so you're a doctor?"

"Of course," I replied.

"If you're really a doctor, how can you possibly believe in ghosts?"

"I don't. If any existed, your charming eyes would drive them all away."

She giggled. "I wish Bill would say things like that to me. All he does is work all day and then he goes to the pub where he spends all his money and doesn't come home until after midnight, completely drunk, drunk. He's an alcoholic with no interest in me at all, at all." She started to weep.

"I felt really lost and alone until I met Antonio. He made me happy again."

"I see," I said, as she continued.

"Then one night while we were in bed I heard the front door opening. It was Bill. He'd come home early, drunk as usual. When Antonio heard Bill coming in, he jumped out of bed, grabbed his clothes and ran naked out of the back door. I felt so awful, I didn't want Antonio to get into any trouble...my drunken husband is such an idiot! Do you know what his reaction was when he saw Antonio's shadow running in the moonlight? He started shouting hysterically to wake me up and told me he'd seen a ghost trying to seduce me and had frightened it away. He stood by the bed with his piggy alcoholic stink and shook me, but I pretended to lie asleep and ignored him. He kept on shouting in a drunken fury; he was so proud that he had chased the ghost away before it took over the whole house. What an idiot!!"

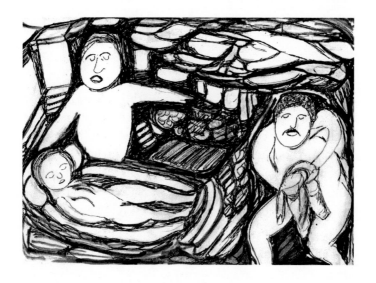

I nodded. "Hmmm…I see…" I murmured as she carried on. "Does he really still want me to believe that our house is haunted by a ghost trying to seduce me?" "Tell me," I replied.

"Is that why he wants you to be Christ and has brought you here? God help him, the poor insecure man. Why does he have to invent such a stupid fantasy and ignore my needs and make you play his stupid game instead of staying home with me to discuss how to solve our problems like normal people? Tell me, doctor - why is he hiding behind ghosts and avoiding having to face reality?"

I was surprised to learn that ghosts are such an important part of English life. I had met a Lebanese ghost in my childhood and was very interested in meeting someone who knew an English ghost, so I could find out whether or not there was any difference between them.

Barry, my exorcist friend in Chelsea, is famous for banishing ghosts with his patented pendulum technique and a radionic black box. Many rich locals employ him to cleanse their mansions. He is so generous with his spiritual skills that he never asks for money. I asked him to teach me about English ghostly culture and maybe even to introduce me to one or two of them. He took me seriously and cheerfully agreed to help me. He invited me to accompany him to the Chelsea Kitchen in Kings Road, his favourite restaurant, where he thought I might find what I was looking for.

While Barry and I were eating our steak and kidney pie, the owner came up to us. I noticed that she was limping and could hardly walk, so I whispered to Barry, "Look, I can help this woman just by touching her hip where it's calcified. By pressing a bit on her hip joint she'll be able to walk properly."

He was intrigued by my suggestion and wanted to see for himself if I could cure her, as I had claimed. He asked the lame woman if she was interested in trying; when she heard I was a doctor she agreed. After two minutes of gentle manipulation, I asked her to walk, which she did without any pain. Amazed and excited, she said, "Look! Fantastic, fantastic! I am cured! I can walk. I was booked to go into hospital next week for a hip replacement. Now I don't need one any more."

People in the restaurant heard what was happening and became very interested, starting to ask me to heal them of their various health problems, so just for fun I touched them for a bit and they enjoyed it. Many were sceptical and started to question me. One elderly gentleman wondered what kind of doctor I was, and asked whether I was a spiritual healer or a magician. "I am a clown doctor," I replied, "I heal by making everyone laugh."

Gossip about what had happened in Chelsea spread quickly and people started looking for me in the cafés and pubs of Kings Road. They wanted to meet me and asked me to give a talk and healing seminar. There was no escaping it, so I accepted their invitation.

We all met on a Saturday afternoon at a nearby church hall, where I introduced myself to more than fifty people. As soon as I invited members of the audience to come forward for healing, a young man came up to me in a wheelchair. His face was joyful and his eyes full of his confidence in life. I asked him to tell me about his spinal injury.

"I was a paratrooper in the Falklands war. I made a bad parachute landing there and broke my spine."

"What do you feel?" I asked.

"When my doctor told me I wouldn't be able to walk again I felt pretty bad, but I've come to terms with it. I spent a lot of time meditating on my situation and realised I needed to get out there to help others. In fact, I'm making more of a contribution now than when I was only a war hero! To be completely frank, I only came here because a friend of mine spoke very highly of you. I'm not interested in being cured, I'm happy with my situation. I travel around the world giving talks to help other disabled people by encouraging them to become as positive about life as I am." He raised his head, turned away from me and quickly wheeled himself back to the audience.

Another young man walked up to me, supporting himself on crutches. He asked me to help his multiple sclerosis, but I saw how difficult it would be for him to accept his situation. "Why are you so frustrated? Others like you are able to cope and enjoy happy, productive lives" I told him.

"How can you say that? Have you any idea what it feels like to be disabled?" he replied indignantly. Pointing towards the paratrooper, I told him, "There's your example, ask him. He's on a wheelchair and hasn't lost his happiness. He's a hero, be more like him - you could learn a lot from his example."

"Thanks very much, I'm OK. The problem is my MS, not me," he said, baring his teeth in an artificial smile. Pursing his lips, he began to move towards the exit, leaving his crutches behind.

Some people in the audience enjoyed watching his pent-up anger and tension, and started to titter and snigger. As he was walking through the door, a fat man with a red face shouted out after him, "Oi! Don't forget to take your crutches with you, mate!"

I made lots of strange and interesting friends in London. One rainy day I went to consult an English clairvoyant I knew about. I thought talking with him would be fun. He would stimulate my imagination and encourage me with new ideas for my life.

As soon as we met he started to tell me all about myself. Although he had no idea whom I was, he described my accomplishments over the previous twenty years with amazing accuracy and explained to me how I go from place to place on a mission to bring a cultural message of healing to the world.

My ears pricked up with interest when I heard his words. I asked him why I had to live such a frustrating and random life instead of settling down in one place like any successful doctor, enjoying a life of luxury surrounded by friends and a loving family. He replied that it was my destiny to live this way because in a past life I had been Cadmus, the prince who left his kingdom behind and sailed away to help humanity.

I don't know what reincarnation is all about, but was fascinated to know what it would be like to live like Prince Cadmus. It felt good to identify myself with him, and I did so all too easily! I liked the idea of having been an ancient Phoenician prince and was intrigued to know more about him. Perhaps his story would give me some idea of how to structure my life and clear my mind of confusion.

I began to research Cadmus, but what I read about him described him as a legendary figure and I couldn't feel any connection with him. I needed to find someone doing historical research to tell me more. Remembering my old Lebanese writer friends, May and Alfred Murr, the top historians of the Phoenician era, I went to visit them in Beirut to learn about their most recent research on Cadmus.

May told me that the ancient Greeks revered him as a deity, though in reality he was a human being. He left his Phoenician Lebanese homeland just as I had, carrying a cultural message for humanity. I was fascinated to find out that Cadmus had been a man like me, and I wanted to be him.

"Thank you so much for your support and appreciation" I said to May. "I am privileged to hear what you are telling me. You are the only person in the world who has fully documented our Phoenician history, and I'm hungry to know more about Cadmus so that I can learn from his example.."

"My dear Hakim [doctor]," May replied, "the story of European civilisation begins with the Phoenician prince Cadmus, son of Ahiram, king of Tyre. His father sent him with a fleet across the Mediterranean to rescue his sister Europa, who according to legend was kidnapped by Zeus in the form of a bull. In fact, she had been abducted from the palace beach by naval raiders and the Zeus story was invented to protect royal honour. Cadmus sailed with his two brothers and his fleet all around the Greek islands looking for his sister. In the end, he found her living like a queen, safe, happy and surrounded by love amongst the Greek island royalty. Seeing his sister's happiness, the prince defied his father and abandoned his mission of vengeance to occupy the Greek islands by force and return home with

Europa. He laid down his arms and started to teach the tribes the alphabet. There he met and married the beautiful Harmonia and started to introduce civilisation to the Greek tribes. Cadmus built Athens and the Acropolis. He also created Cadmea, a citadel in Thebes where he gathered talented people to work together. Cadmea is named after Cadmus. It was the first academy, from which arose the dawn of European civilisation."

It was fascinating to hear May describe how Cadmus was one of the pioneers of civilisation and that his message was one of compassion, peace and high culture. I started to feel the spirit of Cadmus growing within myself. Whenever I heard anything about him my heart leapt for joy. I fell in love with the man who left behind him all his royal authority and became a true human being, with a great heart as well as a great mind.

Following in his footsteps from our old city of Tyre to Athens, I went to Plaka, where I sat down in a small back street café. My heart danced with happiness to feel the noble spirit of Cadmus everywhere I looked. As I sipped my coffee and gazed at the Acropolis, a soft wind rose up from the dawn of antiquity to caress my face. I fell into ecstasy and rushed to climb up to the ancient temple. I felt a silent welcome from the spirit of the great master, as if every stone of his Acropolis was speaking to me. I stayed there connected with him all night in deep meditation.

I left Athens and continued on my way to Theban Cadmea. As soon as I arrived there and my eyes fell on the ruins, I was filled with the mystical fire of an ancient love. Tears rolled down my cheeks, releasing my pent-up frustrations and driving away all confusion. I fell to my knees and felt a warm fatherly hand holding me. I had been like a child lost in the wilderness and now in Cadmea I found myself. Here was my real home. I had returned to my roots. I belonged to every corner of Cadmea. Cadmus had lived there and now he lives within me. I'll listen deeply to his voice and follow it all my life. I left Greece and continued my journey to Romania. I hadn't been in my beloved city of Cluj for several years. She always remembered me as a foreign medical student and a well-known poet in the Romanian language. The city welcomed me back with love, embracing me as someone for whom they had long been waiting. They wanted to collaborate with me and asked how they could support my healing and cultural work, hoping to bring it to their community to help those in need. But how could I help when Romania had not yet recovered from its old Communist trauma, in which the human spirit had been crushed? I couldn't just walk past their trauma with my arms crossed or pretend to be deaf to their cries. How could I kill my feeling and become ruthless? Could I cut myself off from who I am? I felt so frustrated at my helplessness.

I love Romania. She adopted me and taught me medicine when my motherland was crushed by war. What could I do?

Before I went to bed that night I meditated until I fell asleep. I dreamed I was walking through the ancient ruins of Cadmea. A voice behind me called out, "I know who you are, why you're here and what you want." I turned round and asked who it was. The voice replied "Cadmus". I looked again but there was no-one there. Suddenly a tall slender man appeared by my side. "Are you Cadmus?" I asked.

"I am not, only his envoy. I am here to tell you that he is you and you are he."

Suddenly I was walking down an old alley. As I turned the corner I saw Cadmus waving his rod at an engraved tablet on the wall. He was teaching the alphabet to people sitting around him. I rushed towards him. He handed me his rod, disappeared and I found myself standing in his place pointing the rod at the letters and teaching the alphabet. I looked around and now I was by the statue of Matei Corvin in the centre of Cluj, surrounded by Clujeans. There were my friends Delia, her husband Ovidiu and Fanel.

A knock at the door awoke me from my dream. I looked around and found myself in bed at my friend Ovidiu's house. He was in my room telling me that my lawyer friend Fanel had arrived and I left the room to greet him. Ovidiu's mother invited all of us to drink palinca and to eat with it some slanina, the traditional Romanian country food made from smoked salted pork fat and skin. It was Christmas time. The pig had been slaughtered, the table was groaning with food and Fanel and I quickly polished off a whole bottle of palinca. When Delia saw us emptying the bottle in such a good mood she quickly brought us two more.

Feeling much improved, I started to tell Fanel all about my dream. He was thrilled by the news that he was also in it and staggered to his feet, forcing his heavy body to stay upright as he wobbled around the room shouting with excitement, clapping his hands and applauding me with loud bravos. Fuelled by the heat of the palinca and Fanel's enthusiasm I also jumped up, clapping my hands as we reeled around the room together, congratulating myself

115

that my dream was being realised. Delia and Ovidiu smiled with joy and poured out even more palinca.

Following this brilliant meeting we founded the NGO Cadmea of Cluj. It started its work by publishing all my books, which had been censored under Communism. Many young Romanians applauded me and my chest swelled with pride. I continued my exciting life

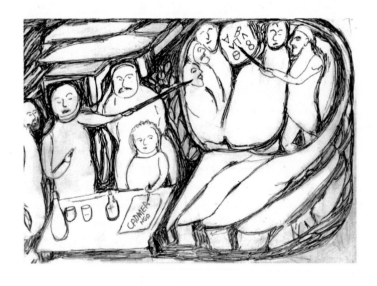

in Romania, spending all my money and enjoying wonderful parties. At every Cadmea meeting I tried to work extra-hard to persuade myself that I really was Cadmus, but always ended up drunk instead. As I wobbled home I often wondered how I had allowed

Cadmus to complicate my life so much. How could I proceed further with my Cadmea?

Well, perhaps all I really needed to do was carry on building it in my brain, discuss it over a drink and get everyone excited!

But, in the end, we decided to start our work by travelling throughout Romania. We journeyed to Bucharest, where I gave many lectures and seminars, and ended up in Moldavia, where I had been invited to give a talk on healing to a thousand people at the Eminescu Theatre in the city of Iaşi.

In the middle of my speech a man in the audience stood up and addressed me in a hoarse voice.

"Doctor, I am diabetic, blind and have gangrene in both feet! I heard you speak on national television this morning. I knew you would be here today and have come to see you with my wife, who has cancer of the oesophagus and my ten-year-old daughter, who was born blind."

I was annoyed with him for interrupting my speech. I walked to the edge of the stage and said gruffly, "I'm not going to give you a private healing session here. Don't interrupt me. How dare you ask me to heal your problem! It's absurd."

"Doctor, I have been trying to track you down for a year. I was lucky to find you here today. I left home with my family at six o'clock this morning and have spent twelve hours getting here. Please be kind enough to spare us a little of your time. I want you to heal us. You are our last resort."

"Too bad, you've come to the wrong person. I don't heal anybody. I can only help you to open your mind so you can heal yourself. That's why I am here, to help everyone to be able to do it and to bring everyone together to create the right atmosphere for group healing."

I turned towards the audience and addressed them in poetic healing language.

"Every word I say is full of vibrations of life energy and inspiration. Every word has behind it a living healing truth. On all my long, hard journey here I have carried my voice to kindle the fire of healing within you. I had to cross many barriers, challenge every obstacle standing in my way and remain vigilant never to allow anyone or anything to compromise my healing message for humanity. What I am now telling you is not based on fantasy nor is it the product of my imagination. It is the fruit of my pure love of life, which I have devoted to the highest principles of our being. The spirit of healing is already incarnated in every word I utter. Let the word knock at the door of your consciousness until it opens to the healing light. By the word we are healed."

The blind, gangrenous old man was deaf to my speech. He was too obsessed with his own problems to listen, as if he was the only person in the audience. He interrupted me again.

"I have left everything behind and came with my whole family especially to meet you so you can cure us of all our sicknesses! I know you can do it, doctor!"

"My dear man, take my advice and let go of your obsession with yourself. Everyone else in the audience is listening to me with detachment, so why can't you? Wait patiently to receive the healing energy you came for, which we are now all creating together. Please feel united with everyone else here and become connected. Harmonise yourself until you are free of all disharmony. Sickness is disharmony, disconnection from the roots of our being and disequilibrium within our natural systems. The moment that self-consciousness tastes harmony, healing occurs. It is spontaneous and dynamic, sometimes even miraculous."

The poor man couldn't understand a word. He was a simple peasant, and all he knew about was feeding his pigs and milking his cows. He paid his doctor's bills with pork, smoked meat and eggs.

"Doctor, give me a prescription. It is now Easter. I have slaughtered a pig and prepared good wine for you."

Everyone in the audience started to laugh at the peasant's efforts to understand my mystical philosophy. The atmosphere started to become as chaotic as a circus. I had to find a way to create a healing psychodrama for the old peasant while also keeping the audience interested and involved. I chose words I knew would have a powerful emotional impact even though he was intellectually baffled.

"My dear man, thank you for coming here. I have no prescription for you and I'm unable to help you as you wish. You have slaughtered your pig in vain. I am not a magician and heal nobody. I only introduce others to the possibility of self-healing. If you have heard of people being healed through meeting me it was always because they found their own inner strength. Since you seem to think that only I can heal your illness I must conclude that you are too weak and feeble to heal yourself."

"Yes I can!" he answered angrily.

I laughed and said, "I don't believe you, prove it!" He looked perplexed and was lost for words as I continued.

"You look as if you're going to die soon. I can't waste any more time talking to you. Come back in two months."

"For God's sake doctor, we can't wait that long. We'll both be dead by then."

"If you want to die go and talk to your priest."

By this time the entire auditorium was in hysterics. Everyone except the old peasant was enjoying my trickster antics and mental judo. I focused my gaze on the poor man.

"If you really have such a heroic wish to heal yourself, you did the right thing by coming here. I think you are incapable of it. The blind who were healed were special people who had God within them, not weaklings like you. As soon as I started to talk to them their sight returned. They came and offered me their spirit of optimistic hope, not a sour face and a basket of eggs!"

The old man rose up from his chair and started to talk with a wild energy, furious at his situation, the humiliation I had heaped on him and the audience's ridicule. He shouted as if a dragon in him had started to breathe the fire of life from his mouth.

"I will show you just how strong I really am. I feel so powerful I'll heal myself this very minute!"

Suddenly I saw his eyes open. His face lit up and he started to cry out for joy.

"Oh my God, I can see! Oh my God, I'm looking at the doctor's face! I can see what he is wearing, even the colour of his clothes. Look! There are his eyes! There is his nose! Holy Jesus, I can feel my legs getting warmer! They're coming back to life! They're not blue any more, they are turning white!"

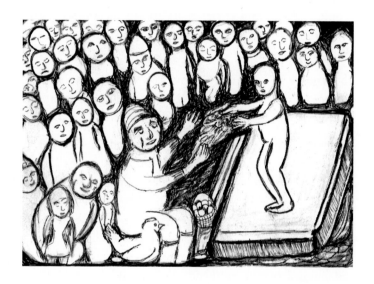

The whole audience became still and silent.

I looked at his legs. It was true, their gangrenous colour had disappeared and they were almost normal. I wasn't surprised because I often see this kind of thing in my everyday life; such phenomena should be seen as natural. Like doubting Thomas, I addressed the man to find out how much he really believed in his own healing powers.

"Are you creating a charade to prove how clever and strong you are? Do you really expect people here to believe your nonsense?"

He glowered at me, raised his legs high in the air, and with tears flowing down his cheeks he cried, "Look, look, look!"

People rushed from their chairs to see the miracle. The hall exploded with deafening applause and loud shouts of "Bravo, bravo, bravo!!"

The energy in the hall intensified, connecting with a universal energy. Everything was transmogrified into a healing pandemonium beyond space and time.

I turned to the old man's wife, who had cancer of the oesophagus and couldn't swallow. As I put my hands on her, he told me not to waste my time because she would soon be dead. Within a short while, her colour improved and she felt fantastic new life energy. I gave her a piece of bread and a glass of water, which she swallowed easily. Then I turned to their blind daughter, sat her on my knee and hugged her to my heart. Entranced, she felt herself melting in the warmth of affection. The old man started to panic when he saw that she wasn't moving. "Doctor, you have killed my daughter."

The audience started to show signs of alarm. Feeling their nervousness, I pinched the little girl. She squeaked and opened her eyes to look up at me and I looked back at her and smiled. Jumping off my knee, she rushed to her mother, crying in amazement, "Mummy, mummy! I can see!" The whole family started to cry with joy and hug each other. I looked at them, saying affectionately "My dear family, now you can see, eat, drink and walk."

Many in the hall were healed without my intervention, simply by being in such a high energy field. A schizophrenic woman started to think and talk normally. Another woman with a large visible uterine fibroid watched it disappear before her eyes. A deaf and dumb child was cured. Silence descended on everyone.

There was nothing left to say or do. I had to go home.

Returning To Myself

I continued my adventures in Romania. All over the country I was warmly welcomed with fantastic hospitality and applauded as a healing superstar. My soul danced with the waves of the Old Danube and sang to the beauty of the famous Romanian folk ballad 'Miorița'. I spent the most beautiful life there, shaded by Carpathian oak trees, singing my poetry with the skylark and the bells. I melted into beauty until I was like the shepherd who offered all his sheep to be slaughtered on the altar of love and all my energy was drained and all my money was gone.

Romania finally had enough of me and I had had enough of her. I left everything behind to continue my journey on my own.

Where to go? What to do? Money all gone, nothing left, not even enough for a ticket out of Romania. If I stayed on there, the time would surely come when I wouldn't even be able to afford to buy a new pair of shoes, and might have to walk around barefoot. I certainly didn't want to end my days in Romania as a shoeless beggar! A meeting with my Cadmean friends over a drink was required to solve my problem.

I invited them to a nice evening party and we danced wildly until everything was clear in my brain. By midnight everything looked very different. The clouds in my head had lifted. All of a sudden the telephone rang. It was my friend the Prince! He was really missing me and our healing sessions. He had already booked a first-class flight the following morning for me to join his party in Geneva.

As soon as I finished my conversation with the Prince, I jumped up excitedly and wobbled around cheerfully kicking all the empty wine bottles until I collapsed to the floor, laughing hysterically and pedalling the air with my legs like a big beetle. My friends thought I had gone totally mad and asked what on earth was going on.

I told them that the Prince had been on the telephone to invite me as his honoured guest and was going to rescue me from Romania. He would reward me handsomely, and I would be able to return as a new person to sponsor my Cadmean activities, with even more fun and wonderful parties.

Full of excitement, my Romanian friends helped me to pack my suitcase, and we continued to enjoy each other's company until the time had come for my departure from Cluj Airport.

When I arrived in Geneva a chauffeur with a black Mercedes limousine was waiting there to take me to the President Wilson Hotel. Everything was so beautiful and peaceful, enjoying walking by the lake and strolling through the back streets of Geneva's Old Town. I stayed for three months and was paid well to enjoy the most luxurious life. I felt wonderful, with no headaches, just enjoying fun and good times with my lovely friend, the Prince.

One afternoon while I was walking by the lake I heard someone in the street calling my name. Looking around,

I saw the smiling face of Wahib, my old Lebanese friend from medical school. We hadn't spoken to each other for sixteen years.

Wahib came from a very poor family and had studied medicine in Romania on a government scholarship. To earn pocket money, he discreetly sold Kent cigarettes and Levi jeans to students in his dormitory. I used to have lots of fun with him and often helped him when he was in need. When I asked Wahib what he was up to in Geneva he laughed, showed me a bank draft for ten million dollars and told me he was in Switzerland on business. Looking closely at me, he could see how carefree I was and invited me to lunch.

While Wahib and I were enjoying some delicious food, he told me that thirteen years earlier his rich uncle in Ghana had died and left him his fortune. He gave up practising medicine and found that it was more comfortable and respectable to work with his money to make even more money. He explained how he had made the shrewd decision to put his assets to work in Romania after the fall of communism, which had multiplied his fortune ten-fold almost overnight. He started showing me a set of business cards, some with the name of his companies around the world and others from his many friends in the Romanian government.

Wahib ended his presentation with a gentle smile and waved his hand at a waiter to order some cognac. What had I done with my life? he asked me – had I made lots of money like he had? I asked him in return how it was possible that he hadn't heard all about me? He must know how respected I am internationally by thousands of people?

I meant to show him that I am much richer than he was and that my wealth was the good energy I had invested in healing people everywhere to make them happy, which is priceless. I gazed into his eyes and calmly told him to look at my face, which would show him how rich I was. But, smiling wryly, he insisted that I was still the same poor guy he knew during our student days.

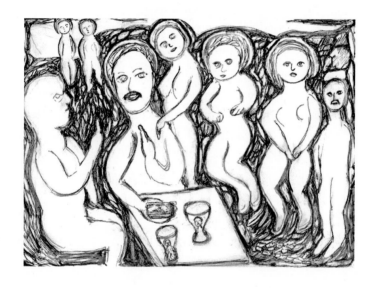

Obviously uninterested in anything I might have to say, he interrupted our conversation to summon one of his bodyguards and gave him ten thousand Swiss francs, ordering him to leave at once to buy two silver-gilt cups. Then he made a phone call to invite three young women from a night club to keep him company that night and told me that I could have one of them if I liked.

I tried to explain that his offer might work for him but not me, but he interrupted me yet again, straightened his head and stared at me with a fixed grin, wagging his finger under my nose. He ordered the other bodyguard to hire two more young women to join him next morning in his private jet.

"All right!" he said. "Did you just see that? This is me. Now you can see how I'm much more than you thought. What about you? Who are you, really?"

I answered him in very few words, flapping and clapping my hands in his face. "I'm also more than you thought. I'm a prince! I'm a great prince, welcomed by the greatest people you've ever heard of. I'm the true prince of all the richness and beauty in the world!"

Irritably, he replied "You're poor and always will be poor. Here's a little gift for you of three thousand Swiss Francs - you look as if you could use it."

I grabbed his money with a laugh. Even a feather from a pigeon's wing can sometimes be a blessing!

That evening I went to the Prince's villa to treat his foot, which had chronic calcification and atrophied tissue damage from a car accident. I'd been treating him regularly for many years and we had become good friends. Sometimes we spent months together travelling around the world. My Prince had special respect for me. I loved him, and was always able to relieve his pain quickly and resolve his health problems when no one else could.

After chatting together for a bit, he asked me to get ready to accompany him to an important reception attended by top business and diplomatic figures. I had to look elegant for the soirée, so he gave me ten thousand Swiss francs to go shopping.

Next day I went out and bought myself a dark grey double-breasted Brioni suit with two Brioni shirts and ties, as well as a pair of black crocodile shoes from John Lobb. I returned to my hotel suite to put on my new clothes and went like a happy child to show myself to my Prince. He was very impressed by my taste and style and told me to be ready to leave with him for the reception in two hours. We had to be there by 7 o'clock. When I said that I would prefer to walk and meet him there, he smiled and told me not to get lost, like the time I strayed over the border into France and had to be rescued.

As I walked across the park I suddenly started to run as if I was a child in the woods again. Looking around, I noticed bunches of green walnuts hanging from an old tree. Their husks were already cracking. I have always been obsessed with eating nuts while they are still white, but the nuts in the park were out of my reach. I had to get at them by any means and tried to climb the tree, but it was too high for me. I looked around for a stone or a piece of wood to throw at the nuts and knock them down from the tree, but couldn't find any.

My craving for nuts made me forget completely that I was an elegant gentleman en route to a VIP reception and my true peasant spirit burst through. I suddenly had a genius idea! I tore the Lobb shoe from my left foot and threw it at a bunch of nuts, aiming well and hitting them squarely, but they stubbornly refused to fall. The shoe remained hanging in the branches, and all I now needed to do was knock down both nuts and left shoe with my right one. I removed it confidently from my foot, took a deep breath and hurled it into the tree. My second Lobb crocodile shoe flew like an eagle and was reunited with its brother, high above me in the old branches.

Omigod! My shoes were gone, dusk was falling and there was no hope of getting them back. To hell with those bloody nuts! Now there was no way for me to attend the reception, shoeless and in my socks. It was getting darker, too late to go home for another pair of shoes and still arrive in time. I'm so unlucky! However others may try to civilise and elevate me I'll always be a stupid fool. I'd lost my shoes, missed my important meeting and had to go home barefoot. The tail of my mind cannot be straightened. Food should be given to someone with teeth to eat it, not an idiot like me. I deserve everything that happens to me.

Those lovely nuts brought me nothing but misfortune. Instead of going like a king to be honoured at a great reception, I ended up trudging home like a shoeless old beggar to bury my frustrated head in a soft pillow.

Next day the Prince asked me why I wasn't at the reception. When I told him about my adventure with the nuts he burst out laughing and couldn't stop. He was so amused by it that he asked me to stay and travel with him, to meet his friends and tell them my nutty story.

So we flew together in his private jet to Paris for a meeting with the President. Upon our landing, a lady in a red coat came to the plane to welcome us and a beautiful red carpet was rolled out, which I was careful not to step on.

As I walked respectfully around it, the Prince watched in amusement and told me with a laugh that the red carpet was there specially for us to walk on.

In Paris I stayed at the Hotel George V, where I enjoyed many days of grand living. Next week we went on to Monte Carlo, where a suite awaited me at the luxurious Hotel de Paris. In the evenings I spent most of my time watching the Prince playing roulette, while during the day I accompanied him all along the Cote d'Azur, visiting many beautiful places in his luxury Maybach limousine.

We continued our journey on his superyacht to Porto Cervo in Sardinia. It was a beautiful sunny day and the sea was as smooth as silk, so I climbed to the upper deck to enjoy the warm sunshine. As the boat left the shore I was fascinated by the beauty of the Alpine landscape and the Cote d'Azur. Passing close to the Corsican shore, I watched the people on the beach through a telescope and my gaze was suddenly drawn to the golden hair of a woman lying there.

She looked like Emma, my former girlfriend from London. I wondered where she was and telephoned her out of curiosity. She was glad to hear my voice and asked me where I was speaking from. When I said that I was standing on the deck of my friend the Prince's yacht passing Corsica, she laughed and told me that she was also in Corsica, lying on the beach looking at a huge yacht passing close to the shore.

"Is that you Rached? The tall bald man standing on the deck holding a telescope?"

"Is that you, Emma? The lovely woman with golden hair on the shore waving her hands in the air?" I replied in turn.

"Yes, it's me, Emma!"

"And it's me too, your crazy old friend Rached!" I laughed. "How amazing!" we shouted cheerfully, waving until we lost sight of each other.

Our yacht arrived at Porto Cervo in the evening, where there were many people waiting for the Prince's arrival. A Rolls-Royce took me to my suite in the most expensive and luxurious hotel and I was offered all the pleasures of life in Costa Smeralda at the best clubs and restaurants. By the end of the week I was totally fed up with so much luxury and couldn't stand any more. I'd had enough.

One morning I woke up feeling uncomfortable, as if a heavy stone was pressing on my chest. I needed to escape to a free and open space, to a wilderness, to my Wilderness. Barefoot, wearing only swimming shorts, I ran downstairs, rushed through the lobby heedless of all the smart people around me and fled from the hotel. Crossing the road like a wild animal, I clambered up a steep hill to the woods leading down to the seashore. No-one was there but me. I galloped along the water's edge shouting angrily at the top of my voice and giving vent to my suffocating frustration. I danced, I sang, I shouted, I roared and howled with craziness, wanting to get back my freedom to be a wild man. I collapsed onto the beach with waves breaking over my head. Miserable, muddy, badly burned by the sun, talking loudly to myself, I struggled to my feet with my whole body shaking uncontrollably and rushed down the road as hot asphalt scorched my bare soles.

A caravan of cars passed me by. One of them stopped and someone shouted out of the window, "What's the matter with you? What are you doing here? You look terrible. Get into the car!"

I looked round and saw it was the Prince.

Calming myself down, to show my Prince that all I was doing was having a bit of fun, I apologised for my muddy appearance and told him I couldn't get into the car because I would dirty the seats. He laughed and told me not to worry but get in anyway, so I sat down next to him with bits of dried mud falling from me onto the white suede seat of his Maybach.

He asked me again what the matter was. Why was I acting so weirdly, wandering about alone in such a wild area without my driver or even a bodyguard? I looked like a lost shoeless vagabond, not someone who had been his guest enjoying the good life.

Grateful for all his kindness and generosity, I thanked him and explained that I must have been born for hardship. I couldn't understand why I had quickly become tired of so much elegant luxury. Was it because I loved the wilderness and always wanted to return to it to enjoy freedom?

The Prince listened quietly. His eyes filled with tears and he smiled. "I wish I could be more like you," he said. "It was my destiny to be born into such a world. I'm trapped in it and know no other way. All that matters is the love we share with each other. Whatever we give each other is given out of love. Thank you with all my heart. Never change; always stay exactly as you are."

I decided to leave all the luxury and beauty of Sardinia behind me. But where to go? I wasn't going back to live in Romania, nor in Lebanon. I had to settle down somewhere to enjoy a simple life and let Lebanon and Romania come to me, not me to them. The mountain had to come to

Moses, not Moses to the mountain, but first I had to find the right place to live.

Was there anywhere in the world where my eccentric personality would be accepted? With all the chaos I create, where could I live like a normal human being? What about England? Many people even weirder than me live there happily. London's climate can tolerate people like me and would suit me well.

What a great idea! Now that I was able to afford to live in the best part of Central London I would become a proper English gentleman. London was where I belonged. I had already received permission from the British authorities to live permanently in the United Kingdom, so why not leave everything behind for the last time and emigrate to London?

So I left Sardinia. As soon as I arrived in London, I moved into a luxury flat near Sloane Square, Harrods and Hyde Park to enjoy a quiet life. It was lovely to be in Chelsea, spending my money in its cafés and meeting other free spirits without ever having to worry about anything. I had to learn how to relax and keep stress and tension at bay. No need to work any more! I was fed up with having to communicate emotionally with my patients to cure them and had had quite enough of sick people's mentality. I needed to slow down and live comfortably, so the British way of life was ideal for me. All I had to do was discuss the weather, go for walks, read the newspapers and visit the pub every day.

This wonderful English life soon tamed me and I became a perfectly quiet and peaceful chap until I got bored. I needed to communicate emotionally with someone. People in England don't like emotional communication and I

134

needed a friend. Maybe having a dog would meet my need. An English dog or even a cat might alleviate my boredom. Pets are the only ones who can tolerate my moodiness. They are always lovely and cute. Wouldn't it be great to have a Labrador? I heard how intelligent and emotionally flexible they are. I really wanted an intelligent and tolerant being to talk to who would understand me.

Having a dog was definitely the answer. I have had many deep friendships with dogs since childhood; we speak the same language.

It was warm and sunny, the first beautiful day of summer. The sun hadn't shone for a long time, so I packed some smoked salmon for a picnic in Hyde Park. On my way, I felt a lot of tension in my chest and needed to talk to somebody. But to whom? There was no-one to talk to so I started to talk to myself in a loud voice and people gave me strange looks.

Maybe they thought that I was just another poor foreign lunatic. I had to be careful not to give English people the wrong impression, and felt more than ever that I had to get a dog as soon as possible. If I had a dog to walk with, everyone would naturally think that I was talking to him and I could babble away to myself freely. I suddenly remembered the time in my childhood when I used to talk with animals.

My best friend was my lovely dog Ruroo, who had once saved my life. Every morning as a child I used to walk for half an hour to my village school. My mother always put a big sandwich in my school bag to take with me. On my way to school I met a spotted dog and we became great friends. He waited there for me every day. I named him

Ruroo. He loved me, I loved him and I always shared my sandwich with him. When my mother found out that her food was going to the dog she beat me, but I went on sharing it with Ruroo anyway.

A year passed and Ruroo disappeared. He wasn't meeting me on my way to school any more. One day while I was wandering through the woods a pack of wild dogs attacked me and were about to tear me to pieces. I panicked: my end had come.

I noticed a spotted dog amongst them which looked like Ruroo. He was preparing to attack me with the rest of them. In despair I cried out, "Rurooo, Ruroo, Ruroo, my friend, rescue me!"

The spotted dog pricked up his ears, threw himself at me in front of the pack, wagging his tail, and turned to confront the other dogs, baring his teeth and snarling to tell them that I belonged to him. The rest of the pack suddenly lowered their heads in confusion and started to back away silently. They turned their backs on Ruroo and me and slunk off furtively. Ruroo jumped up at me and I hugged him with tears of joy. I took him home with me and introduced him to my family.

Arriving in Hyde Park, I started to enjoy eating my smoked salmon picnic under my favourite horse chestnut tree. A black Labrador dog smelled the fish and crept up behind me to steal it. I was so hungry and absorbed that I paid no attention to him, but he wouldn't leave me alone and kept trying to get at my food. I shouted at the dog, gave him a mean and sour look and turned my back on him, frustrating him so much that he went round the tree to raise his leg and pee all over me. I rushed away in disgust to wash my face in the nearby Serpentine and the dog took my place and ate my food.

When his owner saw him eating my lunch he thought I had given it to him and came up to me in a rage. He sternly admonished me, telling me that his dog was on a restricted diet and I was ruining him by allowing him to eat the wrong food. But I had never invited his dog to join me for lunch, I replied indignantly. On the contrary, I turned him away, but he had obviously been so badly trained that he had peed on me and needed to be punished.

The dog's owner replied coldly that there was nothing wrong with his dog, who had behaved quite normally. When I asked him to explain what was normal about his dog's bad behaviour, the man replied that he was upset by my negativity and his correct answer to it had been to pee on me and eat my food.

The dog was right. I shouldn't have shouted at him. It was unkind of me and I could have been gentler. He reminded me of my old frustration at the many people in my life who had stolen from me or taken advantage of me in some other way. That's why I'd reacted to him with such unnecessary anger. Maybe he peed on me to heal me. Anger deserves such therapy.

On the way home from Hyde Park I started to chatter to myself again. Maybe having a dog would be too much right now. Better start off with a cat and get the dog later. My smart friend Sir Tom came into my mind. I hadn't seen or heard from him for over two years. He owns a very beautiful cat. I wish I had one just like his. I'll visit him and ask him where I can buy such a cat and how to bring her up as he did.

Tom lives round the corner from me in Cadogan Square in a big house with many servants. He is so rich that he has never had any need to work and lives such a comfortable life with his family. Their only interest is shopping, giving dinner parties for their friends and elegant gossip. I often dreamed of being like him one day, being rich with no worries and a beautiful cat.

I knew the history of his cat, and I liked the elegant way Tom had brought her up. He had told me that the cat originally belonged to a poor country person and was raised in a rural area where she had to survive by hunting birds and mice. Tom treated her like a member of the family, educating her to behave like a civilised human being, washing and perfuming her every day and feeding her rich food. His family taught her their way of life, how to enjoy the company of visitors, go to bed at a fixed time, and when and how to eat her meals.

That was exactly the type of cat I had been longing for. If I found one I would bring her up to be just like Tom's cat. His house was on my way home, so I passed by hoping to find him in. I missed both Tom and his cat. I rang his doorbell and the butler opened the door. Tom was surprised and pleased to see me after so long, and led me upstairs to the drawing room.

I wondered where his cat was. She used to welcome me as soon I came into the house, purring and rubbing herself against my legs. We sat down and the butler brought a bottle of chilled champagne and two glasses. As we toasted each other, I asked Tom where Wilhelmina the cat was. I missed her and wanted to talk and play with her. Tears welled up in his eyes and he started to tell me a sad story. I listened sympathetically for half an hour, then said goodbye and went home.

That night, I couldn't sleep for thinking about what had happened to the poor, beautiful cat. Living such a luxurious life, Wilhelmina had eventually become fat and lazy and lost her natural instincts. Everything was so easily available to her that she started to be as bored and depressed as everyone else in the family, with nowhere to go and nothing to do. The cat and her family had lost any stimulus or even the slightest stress to motivate them. She became passive, repressed and almost dead emotionally; sweet, polite and docile, with no interest in hunting and killing. She was completely tame and could only communicate in a low, sweet voice, lounging about all day in the drawing room with her owners and relaxing in a bespoke mink-lined Scandinavian meditation basket, as if she was the first lady of the house.

The previous winter something terrible had happened. A little field mouse came to live in Tom's house and the bored Wilhelmina was happy to meet a new playmate. She welcomed the little mouse as an honoured guest and invited it to play her favourite game with a ball of silk thread.

Unfortunately for the kind and gentle cat, the field mouse was uneducated and still had its original wild nature. He didn't understand what the cat was trying to tell him and thought his life was in danger. Seeing no escape, he sank his teeth into the cat's forepaw and bit into it aggressively.

The cat, having lost her natural instinct to kill, had no idea what to do. She ran away from the mouse and hid in her mink-lined basket, nursing her wound. She soon collapsed from tetanus and was dead within the hour.

Her original nature had been perverted and her immune system corrupted. Civilisation killed the cat.

I think I've had enough. I'll go on living happily in London as I am, grateful for everything I've been through in life. There is no need for me to do more than I have already done or to have more than I already have.

Peace is all I need.

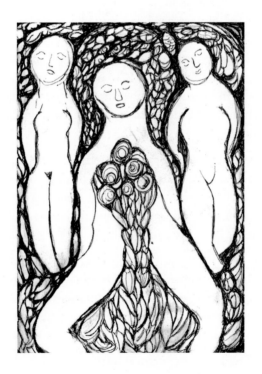

Every Malady Has a Remedy

Over the last twenty-five years I have been able to heal many patients who came to me with incurable medical conditions. I treated them successfully and without risk by adding to my orthodox practice innovative medical skills, new diagnostic methods and new therapeutic approaches. I explored the human condition underlying disease pathology and treated each patient as a unique case, studying all the objective morphological and physiological signs and symptoms of the pathology of his or her illness, as well as subjective ones that manifest psychosomatically and are specific to the individual.

In order to heal my patients, I found that it was important to understand and feel them as human beings rather than treating them mechanistically, as if they were simple biological organisms.

I always begin a medical interview by discussing the patient's previous medical tests and treatments, why they were unsuccessful and what more could have been done. Only when they are willing to admit that conventional medicine is no longer able to help them do I feel free to introduce my new methods and therapeutic techniques. To be able to heal my patients I work on their minds to open them to my new approach, as well as on myself to become full of compassion and creative inspiration. I have to approach each case in a state of harmony, detached within myself, free from tension, obsession, frustration or anxiety. I need to be selfless and inwardly relaxed in order to relax others.

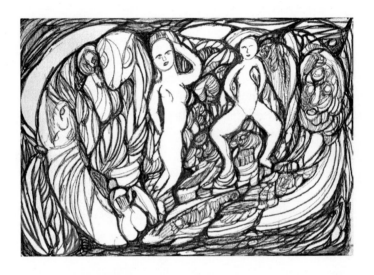

Whenever a patient comes for a session with sickness caused by a physical problem, as in most sport injuries, neuromuscular disorders and so on, I manipulate their muscles, ligaments, joints and nerves. Once my therapy has produced good results, I still have to work to change their minds to help them to acknowledge that they are no longer sick. Recovering from physical illness while the mind still has thoughts of illness can be temporary and the health problem may come back. In cases of chronic illness patients need time to become convinced that they really are cured. They are fully healed only when they have seen the positive results for themselves and fully recognise that they are well and no longer sick.

Sam's Case

Sam, a 35-year-old Londoner originally from Lebanon, came to see me one afternoon for a consultation. He had been suffering from back pain for more than five years. His spine was twisted and curved to the right. After examining him, I offered to treat his back.

Within half an hour of deep tissue massage he was able to stand up perfectly straight and without pain, but when I asked him whether my session had brought any improvement he replied that nothing had changed - his back was still the same as before. Although I told him to look in the mirror to see how straight his back now was, he replied that my therapy hadn't worked and had brought him no results. He seemed to be looking through the same old eyes with which he had first met me. I tried once again to convince him that his back was cured, but he went on denying it.

Sam probably wasn't lying. He was still living in the past when his back was bent and didn't know how to live in the present in which I had straightened it. He was truly unable to see what was happening to him. When I looked into his eyes they were soft and friendly, without the slightest trace of deceptiveness.

I felt that the memory of his illness was still in his brain and needed to be dissolved. Somewhere in his neurons there still lurked an encoded program of his old back problem, overshadowing his mind. Living with back trouble for five years had encoded a pathological neural program in his brain. It wasn't enough for Sam's body to be cured; his mind also needed curing. He had to rewire his neurons with a new program of the healing I'd already done for his back. I had somehow to make him aware that my half-hour treatment had resolved his five-year problem.

I continued my treatment by helping him to free his mind of the negative emotions distorting his perception so he could see that his back was back to normal. Using touch, speech and psychodrama, I stimulated all his energy points to activate a neurochemical process which would encode in his consciousness the new healing reality. As Sam started to feel more emotionally secure he became able to see himself standing up straight and was astonished. Happy and amazed, he looked at me and asked, "Doctor, how long will my back stay straight?"

"That's up to you," I answered with a laugh. "Tell me how many years' guarantee you'd like and I'll write you one."

The Healing Relationship

Healing can't happen until one is free of negative emotions. The essential role of the therapist is to create the right conditions for this to occur. Whenever we are insecure, fearful, defensive or anxious the body secretes stress hormones which open the way to sickness. When we become peaceful and harmonious the brain secretes neurotransmitters which stimulate a process of neuroplasticity to activate the healing system within the body.

I have to find a way to communicate with each patient in his or her own personal language. It doesn't matter whether or not they understand the process as long as they are trusting, relaxed and have the security and confidence for the healing process to occur. I often have to fit myself into the mental framework of others, avoiding argument so as not to create any misunderstanding which might disturb our communication and become an obstacle to healing. I usually don't even try to explain to my patients my unusual healing work in words, leaving them to experience and respond to it in their own way.

Healing speaks for itself. Sometimes the mind can't readily absorb a healing reality beyond its understanding and prefers to stay secure within its limitations. I don't allow myself to impose on anyone by giving them more than they ask for or need to know, so as to avoid negatively affecting our healing relationship. I simply relate harmonically to the uniqueness of each patient to create the right healing chemistry.

Most importantly, the chemistry of relationship with my patient gives good healing results only when it is based on a spirit of trust without expectation. My patients' spirit of confidence and trust often helps me to end many years of suffering. They are cured quickly and are grateful, even though they have no idea how their healing might have been accomplished.

The Chemistry of Healing

After a lifetime of extensive clinical experience involving many thousands of patients, I have found that whenever there is good chemistry between me and my patient healing can occur in the best way. The classical medical approach of diagnosis and treatment alone is insufficient. There also needs to be empathy and a deep human touch for me to cure my patients. My healing occur as inspiration and revelation when my relationship with them becomes truly free, full of peace and beyond all boundaries. I struggle with each patient to build a special world of connectedness and unconditional love to reveal in him or her the creative possibility of self-healing.

At this point the patient suddenly feels free, relaxed and full of hope, their face illuminated with ecstasy as the spirit of healing brings inner joy. There is a power of spiritual love within the healing relationship that brings inner security and deep relaxation, dissolving all negative stress. Human consciousness expands into a universe of beauty beyond space and time where the laws of physics can be challenged and the body can reverse its pathology to cure itself.

The chemistry of relationship has a vital role in curing illness. I'm always working on myself to become lively, selfless and harmonious within to inspire my patients with positive healing energy. Only through compassion, affection and detached intimacy can their consciousness shift to transform their frustration, fear, grief and insecurity into joy, surrender and inner peace. They become ecstatically connected with their beautiful interior world, which is often reflected in the spontaneous disappearance of their illness. When there is this unconditional healing intimacy between me and a patient, perhaps our bodies release chemicals of empathy such as oxytocin, as occurs between lovers or between a mother and her child. These chemicals may act as neurotransmitters to form a neural web which encodes a program of healing information to instruct the body to cure itself.

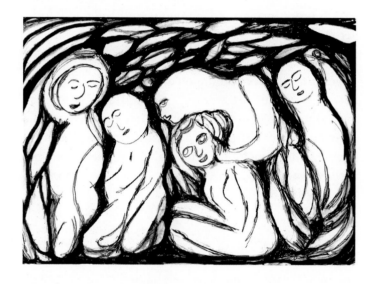

Mrs B's Case

Mrs B, a woman with terminal cancer, was told she had only two months left to live. Like anyone, she was unable to cope with the shocking news. From the moment we met I felt we had good healing chemistry and empathy. I noticed that I was in an unusually positive mood, able to listen to her with all my heart, and she also responded well to me. I wanted to inspire her to be healed by letting go of all her dark thoughts and fully accepting her situation.

I had to work on her mind, firstly to revoke the sentence of death her doctor had imposed on her, and secondly to liberate her from her worries, fears and anxieties. Later on, I would freely inspire her with more compassion and affection to give her greater emotional security. I wanted her to fall in love with herself, even with the cancer within her body, and to become totally connected within in full harmony and inner peace.

My therapeutic scheme was to free her of negative emotions which might have provoked in her the production of stress hormones such as cortisol, weakening her immune system. Negative emotions might indirectly promote oxidative stress, with an increase in free radicals which damage tumour-suppressor genes like p53, making it unable to control cellular growth or prevent cancer cell multiplication. I would employ my unorthodox medical-spiritual approach to inspire her non-verbally, enabling her to transform negative emotions (distress), mental fears and anxieties to the positive emotions (eustress) of inner security, ecstatic love for herself and inner peace. Under these new conditions consciousness undergoes a perceptual shift, automatically triggering neurotransmitters to stimulate the neurons to rewire themselves within a web encoded with self-healing information.

This process is essentially collaborative and requires the full participation of the patient's will and awareness to be healed

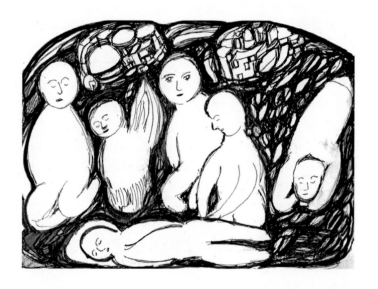

by any means possible. Mrs B had to live fully believing in her healing ability in order to create within her brain the healing information appropriate to her case, transcribed in messenger proteins carried to the chromosomes to switch on certain genes to instruct the body to heal itself. She needed to acknowledge that cancer is neither a death sentence nor a foreign invader of the body. It should be treated with harmonising love and understanding, not with any type of clinical aggression.

Cancer cells are ageless. They are part of our bodies; we are born with their stem cells and they live in us under a system of harmonic control and cellular homeostasis. Cancer originates from any disharmony or disorder which disrupts cellular homeostasis. Disequilibrium can originate at any level – physical, mental, emotional, social, spiritual – negatively impacting through an individual's relationships within himself and with others to increase the risk of cancer. Embryonic cellular memory within the body is affected; cancer stem-like cells develop in a chaotic way and a program of metastasis takes over.

I applied my theory to poor Mrs B by addressing her intellectual obsessions in a manner designed to neutralise them. While she was giving me funny looks, I intentionally bombarded her with complicated theories so as to take her mind off her obsessions, with the intention that a program of self-healing would establish itself and work without interference. I concluded my scientific campaign with a pleasant chat.

"What is going on with you?"

"What is going on? I have stage IV cancer. My doctor told me I will be dead in two months. I won't be spending Christmas with my children this year."

"I see. If what your doctor told you is true there's no point in my trying to heal you. It would be more practical for you to buy a coffin and plan your funeral." She smiled and replied comically.

"Thank you, doctor, that's an excellent idea! Don't forget to invite all your friends to my funeral. I'll make sure we have a wonderful party afterwards."

"Die first and we'll discuss it in detail later."

"Doctor, I'll always enjoy our lovely discussions. We will have lots more parties, even after my funeral. My spirit loves you and I'm sure it will keep on visiting you."

"Then please can you tell me what you think you will lose when you die?"

"I will miss seeing my children," she replied.

"Don't worry. Your children will be fine, they can manage. Just leave them all your possessions and they will be very happy." I asked her again what she thought she would be losing.

"I don't know, tell me." She was lost for words. She already saw herself at her funeral party and going on to meet me afterwards, so she could see that death would not be the end of her. Maybe, by now, she understood deeply that death itself is also part of life.

"I will explain it to you simply," I told her. "All you will lose is your fear of death. Don't wait for your last breath to realise that there is nothing left to fear. Surrender your fear now and peacefully join yourself to the flow of life. You have so many beautiful things to enjoy."

She was filled with inspiration to hear these words. Astonishingly, ten years later she is still alive and enjoying life as a party.

Further Considerations

Can these concepts be developed into a general theory? Were my patients who suffered from advanced cancer cured by my application of the chemistry of therapeutic relationship, or did they just heal themselves through spontaneous remission, which might have happened anyway without my intervention? Perhaps my intervention and our personal chemistry together stimulated the self-healing process.

It is known that spontaneous remission of cancer occurs occasionally with or without medical intervention. Because cancer cells grow chaotically, invading healthy cells and obstructing the body's physiological functions, they can probably also invade each other, blocking their own functions and becoming destroyed in what is known as apoptosis or cellular suicide.

Did my love for those cancer patients who were cured terrify their neoplastic cells sufficiently to persuade them to spread so crazily and chaotically that they ended up committing collective suicide? Is a lack of love an invitation to cancer cells to invade the organism, and is that why only when love is present do they cease their offensive and sue for peace, which can result in spontaneous remission? Does the absence of love play a role in the multiplication and proliferation of cancer cells?

If a lack of love can indeed make someone so emotionally negative that it could provoke cancer cells to proliferate and become aggressive, invading their whole organism, it makes no sense to treat the cancer with aggression instead of love, or to declare war against it using weapons of cellular mass destruction such as chemotherapy and radiotherapy.

Living in fear, emotional repression, insecurity and anxiety releases stress hormones in the body such as cortisol, leading to immunodeficiency and cellular oxidation reactions which can increase the level of oxidants and free radicals. These can then block and paralyse the function of repressor genes such as p53 which control the proliferation of cells to inhibit the growth of tumours.

Most of my cancer patients were apathetic, with a death wish of which they were unaware. This may have been a causative factor in stimulating cancer cells to bring the death which they had unconsciously been seeking. Many cancer patients are unaware of their negative emotions. Perhaps this depression or apathy is born with the person, or perhaps it is caused by past emotional trauma. Depression can turn into an unconscious death wish, or vice versa, and the body may somatise the negative pattern, stimulating cancer stem cells to proliferate and hasten death.

It looks as if whenever there is good chemistry in the therapeutic relationship it can inspire patients to transform negative emotions like fear, which favours the growth of cancer, into positive emotions like love. Through our affectionate therapeutic relationship I inspire them to love life and feel connected to it, to free themselves from emotional insecurity and anxiety and to become full of confidence, hope and pride.

As soon as patients open up, lose their fear and experience compassion, they feel as if something so beautiful is happening within them that it lifts them above all their suffering and misery, bringing joy, ecstasy and surrender. There is a sudden shift in consciousness that transforms the negative emotions of apathy (whether conscious or not), in which one feels that existence has no meaning and is an illusion, into a positive pattern where one sees that the whole world is itself an illusion, the real meaning of which can be found only in the creative life within oneself.

To open up the possibility of healing for cancer patients, their negative emotions need to become positive. In cases when patients present signs of the apathy which often underlies cancer, the healing process has to go through several stages. In each stage there are several emotional phases associated with certain biochemical processes.

In the first stage: the patient's stress hormones such as cortisol are activated. They become emotionally negative and despondent.

In the intermediate stage: the patient's adrenaline becomes more active. They feel anger and pride and are ready to fight for their identity. They feel highly confident and are ready to find a solution to their problem.

In the last stage: the patient starts to feel hopeful and able to struggle to cure the cancer. They feel calm within, as if they are connected to the universe and no longer abandoned by life. They surrender, feeling compassion and a love of life, even ecstasy. Neurotransmitters such as serotonin, dopamine and endorphins activate a mechanism of neuroplasticity, forming a neural web in which a healing program is encoded. This program sends messages for the body to regulate its cellular homeostasis, restoring harmony between the cells to heal itself from cancer.

Classical medical thinking based on aggression rather than compassion must end its war on cancer. Cancer needs to be treated differently: cancer cells are not our enemies; they are born in all of us as stem cells and haven't come from outside to invade us like foreign bodies or biological agents. That is why our immune system may not consider them enemies or try to fight them.

Everyone has cancer cells in the body and can live with them in harmony unless adverse factors provoke the cancer stem-like cells to multiply. In our body there are negative cells which lead to death as well as normal positive healthy cells which nourish life. Life itself is based on the harmonious interaction of opposites, and we need to realise that we exist through the harmony of opposites called death and life. It is normal for our bodies to have cells which carry the message of death, called cancer, to our healthy somatic cells, which carry the message of life.

Cancer therapy should not be based on brutality towards the negative cells (cancer) but should instead work to restore the energetic balance between cells. It looks as if the homeostatic cellular balance is disturbed when normal somatic cells (positive cells) weaken and age and cancer cells (negative cells), which are vital, youthful and ageless, take over and dominate through metastasis. Medicine needs to abandon its aggressive approach through the kind of chemotherapy which destroys not only cancer cells but also healthy cells. Healthy normal cells must not be allowed to become weak, giving cancer cells the opportunity to proliferate and invade.

The right way to help the body to heal itself of cancer is by strengthening its healthy cells, restoring their vitality and bringing them into dynamic equilibrium so as to stimulate the control system which inhibits tumour growth. The human organism is a self-harmonising system which needs to remain stable, enabling opposites to balance each other for our well-being.

Does the chemistry of my therapeutic relationship with cancer patients indirectly stimulate their normal somatic cells to confront the cancerous cells and prevent their infiltration throughout the body? Can the creative love which brings harmony inspire the body to heal itself of cancer?

Healing Chemistry: A Testimonial

Veronica Avalos, a young American woman, was in the final stage of cancer and was not expected to survive for more than a few days. Her friend Kathy invited me to go with her and visit Veronica for a coffee.

Kathy had told me that Veronica had cancer and asked if I would go with her to see her friend. She had previously persuaded Veronica that I was the only person in the world who could help her and to accept my visit.

As soon as I entered Veronica's house, I was surprised to see her lying in bed with an oxygen mask and perfusion bag, unable to breathe and almost suffocating. She was about to die.

I looked into her eyes and felt her suffering. I was deeply moved. I wanted to share her pain and held her in my hands. At least the touch of my hands on her chest and back might help her breathing.

As soon as I laid my hands on her I felt a wonderful warm, peaceful energy flowing through us. I cannot tell the story better than Veronica herself:

"In October 1999 I was diagnosed with Stage IV Non-Hodgkin's Mediastinal Lymphoma with Lung Involvement. It was inoperable and the tumour was connected to my aorta, oesophagus and every major organ in that area.

"My doctors informed me that there was nothing that could be done for me due to the severeness of my illness. All they were offering was hospice care. They said that I would be dead before Christmas. I was devastated and felt cheated by life. I left the hospital about a week later to go home, basically to die. The day I came home Kathy Elden, a good friend of mine, called me and told me that there was this wonderful man she had met that she wanted me to see. She wanted to come over that night and bring him to my house because she felt he could help me. I have never been the type of person who believed in healers, but I knew Kathy had made a great effort to arrange it. I agreed for them to come to my house that night.

"When I first met Rached I wasn't really concentrating on him because I was hooked up to IVs and was using oxygen to breathe and extremely tired. In addition, I was preoccupied with my children's future and trying to figure out what had to be done before I died. Rached spoke to me about the Bible, about Christ and how I should see my illness. He spoke to me for a couple of hours. The main thing I remember of our discussions which I used to help me get through the bad days was that I was not to wage a war against cancer, I was to try to become one with it and live with it. Also, we spoke of the story of when Christ went into the desert for forty days and forty nights with no food or water. After the forty days he began to despair, and that was when Satan came.

"Rached told me to always try to have a positive attitude and be happy because if I began to despair the cancer would take over. There were days that I wanted to die, but Rached's words always came back to me and pulled me through. I always tried to find the positive side of having cancer, something that Rached taught me. My doctors were amazed at my attitude and felt it played an important part in my recovery.

"After Rached and I spoke he told me he was going to show me. I had no idea what he meant. He hugged me very close to his body and I felt very safe and in a state of euphoria. It felt like nothing I have ever experienced before except in Rached's presence. After he finished I vomited, as I did frequently, but this was the first time there was no blood in my vomit. My night nurse was amazed. I was told later that Rached had moved my body into different positions and had pressed hard on a two-day incision that was five inches long. My husband told me he thought I was going to scream, but I just lay there. He also told me Rached healed me for about an hour though I felt that it was a matter of minutes.

"Rached told me that I had to continue Western medical treatment, but that I would live and the cancer would go away. That night was the first night in months that I was able to sleep on my back and to sleep the night through. I had not been able to lie on my back because the tumour weighed heavy on my chest and restricted my breathing. When I went back to the doctors a few days later they were confused at my X-rays. They said that the tumour had shrunk. I knew it was Rached, but the doctors said a lot of different things could have happened. They would not believe in Rached, which angered me.

"I saw Rached a few days after our first meeting and, as before, I felt so much better. Rached told me that he had to leave the country, but that he would be there for me if I needed him. I did survive and fooled all the doctors. The only problem that remained was that my lungs had been very damaged by the cancer and I would have to use oxygen for the rest of my life. My lung capacity was 43%.

"I saw Rached a couple of years after my initial meeting and I had three or four healing sessions with him. It was January. In October of the previous year I had had my latest PFT (Pulmonary Function Test) done and I was still in the low 40s. After my sessions with Rached in January I requested to be retested. My lung capacity had increased to 64%. I now no longer take steroids and do not need oxygen.

"I believe that Rached is truly a man of God and that he was put on this earth to aid people. He works as a tool of Christ, which enables us to heal ourselves. I think that I would not be here to tell my story if it wasn't for Rached. I knew the first night I met him that he was something special. I remember I asked him if I could kiss him on the cheek and knew at that moment that I felt a very pure sense of love for him and that I would never forget him. Rached is my angel on earth and he is never far from my thoughts. Now we keep in touch via the internet and I am always amazed that if I feel down or I am having a problem it seems that I get a note from Rached. He tells me I am in his thoughts and that he always knows how I am doing.

Knowing that makes my life easier. I feel I have God on my side.

Veronica Avalos, Los Angeles March 2006

P.S. "In September 2013, Rached asked me if he could publish my story in his book and I agreed. I can add that I have not had a relapse and am completely healthy and happy."

Healing Chemistry: A Case Study

Sharif was a patient in his forties with hydrocephalus caused by a brain tumour obstructing the cerebral ventricle. He would lose his equilibrium and fall over whenever he tried to walk. The pressure of liquid in his brain had affected his entire nervous system, making his limbs shake continuously. He couldn't see clearly and everything around him looked foggy.

I had heard about his illness. His case looked too difficult and beyond my capacity to cure. How could I possibly have been able to help him? What did using my hands have to do with curing hydrocephalus?

I was in conflict within myself. On one hand, I think like any other medical professional and knew that Sharif's illness was incurable. On the other hand, I felt that he might find a healing power within himself and I could be the catalyst for his healing. Which path should I follow, knowing his life was at risk? I didn't know what to do, and decided to keep him waiting in the hope of eventually seeing me.

I wanted to see Sharif only if I was one hundred percent certain that I could cure him. Who knows whether or not he was looking for a miracle? Was he a sceptic or a perfectionist? What did he expect me to do for him? If my therapy could help him, would he be ready for it? Surely it was better for me not to see him immediately but to wait until he was ready for healing. Why should I risk failure by trying to help him at the wrong time, when his situation was still unclear? Perhaps Sharif might die before then. Should I even think about trying some healing for him now before it was too late, knowing that I would probably fail? But things with Sharif were to turn out differently. The wind does not always blow as the sails wish, but in the end they find the harbour.

One day while I was visiting patients in Bucharest, Delia and Louisa, my two bright young assistants, announced that a new patient called Sharif had arrived and was waiting in the reception room to see me. I was extremely irritated to hear that they had booked an appointment for him without first asking me and told them angrily to invent any excuse to get rid of him because I didn't have the energy or inspiration to handle his case. They just had to tell him politely that I couldn't see him now because he had been booked in by mistake and my schedule was already full. We would put him on the waiting list and try to make another appointment over the next three days while I was in Bucharest. He should go home and wait for me to call him.

The girls went back and told Sharif I was in a bad mood and couldn't see him; if they insisted, Dr Daoud would go crazy. He said he would wait for me in the reception until I was in the mood to see him for a brief consultation and take a quick look at his medical file. They returned and hugged me, telling me they had solved the problem beautifully. Trying to calm me down with her charm, Delia smiled, took my hand with tears in her eyes and said in a soft voice how much she admired what I do for my patients, how beautiful it was to see patients arrive sad and in pain and leave with a smile on their face.

As Delia spoke I felt all my frustration go, leaving me feeling calm yet filled with excitement. She saw the love and humanity shining in my face once again. All my dark thoughts and medical obsessions vanished and I felt the healing power coming back to me. As Delia saw me responding to her words, she put her arms around my neck, looked deeply into my eyes and said, "Do you love me and do you want me to be happy and proud of you?"

"Of course I love you and want you to be happy!" I replied.

"Then you should also be happy to say hello to Sharif. You are going to love meeting him and seeing what a nice, good man he is. He only wants to see you because he has heard what a lovely human being you are, not because you're a doctor and he needs you. How beautiful for you to meet him, whether he is a patient who needs you or not."

"Who is this charming Sharif you are so excited about? Is he your new lover?"

"Of course he is!"

"Who is he? Where is he?" I laughed.

"He's in the reception room. He came this morning and is still waiting outside. I told him you're here and he's waiting for you to say hello whenever you like, if you have time."

I felt trapped by Delia's charm and was torn. Delia's enthusiasm had made me want to meet Sharif as a friend,

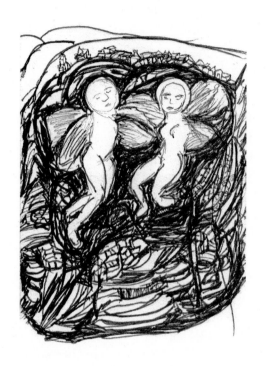

but I didn't want to see him as a patient as his case was so difficult. I started to feel anxious again.

"As soon as I saw Sharif in the reception room this morning," Delia continued, "I felt how special he was! He is so nice, so lovely, such an attractive human being. I love him."

"Do you mean Sharif, the patient with hydrocephalus?"

"Yes I do, I do."

"But we have just escaped from him. Why do we need to discuss him? Let's just enjoy our coffee?"

"He's waiting outside. Offer him one of your lovely smiles and he'll be healed."

"So be it!"

Suddenly I felt an angelic beatitude fill me with inner peace and joy. I felt so beautiful, passionate and excited to see Sharif. No more did I fear his hydrocephalus, my heart became drunk with love and, awakening from beneath the wreckage of my professional frustration, I rushed downstairs to meet him. Delia looked after me in astonishment, calling out after me "Hey, you crazy man, are you trying to escape? Don't forget you're meant to be a doctor. Wait here for your patient and I'll fetch him for you."

Sharif came through the door with a smiling, joyful Delia. As soon as I looked into his eyes a deep serenity came over me. The lovable humility and simplicity of a natural mystic shone from his face. His eyes glistened, inspiring me with his beauty. I saw that his gratitude and surrender had empowered him to face his sickness and become free of any negative emotions. I laid Sharif's head upon my shoulder, feeling the beautiful child in him. My hands flowed over his head, neck and shoulders. Waves of love came to carry us beyond space and time. A great silence filled us.

In spite of his hydrocephalus, Sharif had no negative emotions, no frustration or anxiety. He was full of hope. In his charming simplicity and childlike naiveté, he perceived everything as positive. He was a real spiritual man and within ten minutes of my putting my hands on his head all the cloudiness in his visual field had cleared. His limbs stopped shaking, he regained his balance and was able to walk steadily. Leaving the room excitedly, he ran up and down the stairs full of joy.

Within three days Sharif was able to drive a car again, gaining so much confidence that after only one week he drove all the way from Bucharest to Rome to visit his daughter. A month later his MRI scan showed that the tumour had shrunk and was no longer obstructing his

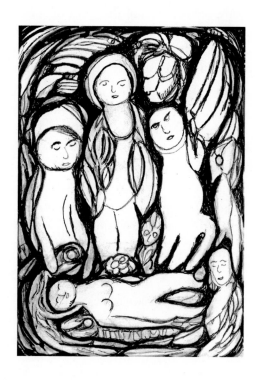

cerebral ventricular foramina. Sharif's cerebrospinal fluid was circulating normally and no longer accumulating to cause hydrocephalus.

Some terminal cancer patients are able to see that their healing lies beyond the physical. They understand that they need to surrender to life and accept their death as part of it. They become able to face it joyfully, grateful for life as it is. Life is more important than healing; even death is a form of healing.

Once a young woman came to me with cancer spread all over her body. She was full of the spirit of surrender and acceptance. We met daily to share beautiful things together, feeling as if time had stopped. She lived in a world of never-ending ecstasy until she died in a state of well-being and joy.

She often told me, "Death is the most important part of life. It's better for me to die healthy than to live sick."

Healing Determination

I neither try to persuade any of my patients about anything nor encourage them to believe in me. I promise them nothing, respecting their freedom to make their own decisions and take full responsibility for their lives. Healing cannot come from outside or be imposed by someone else. My patients have already tried everything, so all that remains for them is to find their own healing solution within. All I can do is to inspire them with enough self-confidence to believe that they deserve to be healed.

Deep within every patient there is an inner knowing calling him to find the right way. My healing duty is to awaken my patients to its voice and my role is to be ready to tune into it. Each patient is original and unique. His or her healing also works in a unique way. I must always be ready to listen with selflessness to my patient's inner healing voice, which will lead me to the right therapeutic approach. The healing has to come from within my patient. My role is to reflect it back, expressing it through my medical skills applied harmoniously to their unique case with all the language and colours of their human individuality. I need to be in deep resonance with my patient's inner reality.

To challenge minds conditioned by the mentality of illness and turn them positive, I have to cooperate with the healer within them, their inner knowing or true consciousness. I have to work with the power within everyone, an enlightened love that guides the healing process. Sometimes it even appears to defy natural law. That is why the deep chemistry of relationship between the patient and me is essential. The body-mind with all its emotions has to be free and open, to reflect in reality the inner will of the patient, giving him or her the right to be healed. I have to create the right atmosphere to be allowed to enter deeply into my patient's heart and soul. I can only do this when I feel the flow of love which takes me beyond myself.

During the healing session, my patient also has to feel free of himself or herself. They need to allow their mind to empty itself of all its past conditions, to live in the healing inspiration of the present with its deep feelings of inner peace.

When I work on my patient I feel as if I am in a trance, drunk with beautiful healing energy. I stop my mind, leaving myself behind to enjoy my work in complete harmony, connected to him or her through my therapeutic touch, speech and gestural language. They feel the flow of love, which carries them beyond space and time to a warm, safe place where all their worries and anxieties are dissipated. Later on, they return to normal consciousness healed like a newborn child re-entering the world.

Being Human to Treat the Human

Seriously ill patients who have lost hope of ever being cured usually come to me only as a last resort. Their ill health has made them apathetic, depressed, anxious, insecure, exhausted, fearful and hopeless. Their emotions have turned negative so that they can defend themselves psychologically. They arrive feeling beaten down and victimised, as if life had treated them unfairly and ruined their chances of happiness. They often believe that I can't really help them, but come anyway because they have nothing better to do. All their hopes of medical salvation have been dashed and they cannot even bear the sight of another doctor. To win their trust and be able to collaborate with them, it is essential for me to introduce myself to them as a fellow human being willing to share their suffering.

When patients feel that they are being treated in a friendly, human way they start to relax and experience their humanity as something quite separate from their sickness. They are able to see their situation more objectively and accept their illnesses as part of life, not as an enemy coming to destroy them.

As soon as someone contacts me with a health problem I open my heart and treat them as a fellow human being, rather than as a client coming to me out of fear and neediness. I provoke them with compassion so as to free them from the mentality of sickness with which nearly all patients are burdened. I communicate with them heart to heart, and healing starts in the light of our creative positive relationship.

My therapeutic work always needs to create a positive atmosphere. During our healing session, my patients forget that they are ill and I also forget that I am a doctor. All masks have to fall away; illness is one of them. Whenever someone enters my practice looking serious and troubled at the thought of having to visit yet another doctor, I dislike being made to feel as if I ought to behave like a typical medical expert in his clinic. I will do anything to break such an authoritarian way of thinking.

Why should I practise medicine like a prosecutor looking for diseases with which to condemn and victimise patients, manipulating them through fear? I refuse to be a judge or executioner delivering sentence on my seriously ill patients and prefer to relate to them as an artist using his creativity to inspire healing and lift them above their misery.

Sometimes I even play the fool to decondition their minds from the seriousness of their illness. I never bother about how I first appear to my patients; I just need to act appropriately to mirror their reality and create good relationships through which the healing process can occur.

On occasion a patient has come into my clinic and, seeing me open the door to him in casual clothes, even asked me where the doctor was. Whenever this happens, I offer him a chair and say the doctor is on his way. I may sit chatting with him in the reception room until he is so relaxed that he is no longer preoccupied with his patient status and his fears dissipate. Only then do I introduce myself as the doctor; sometimes they think I am joking.

Once I even told a new patient that Dr. Daoud had died. He was so upset at the sad news that the famous miracle worker was no longer in the world to help him and all afflicted sufferers that we both burst into tears. Only after several minutes of heartfelt weeping was I able to bring him the happy news that Dr. Daoud had returned to life and was sitting beside him. His back pain immediately vanished.

Having a belief system can give some patients a certain emotional security and strength to cope with their anxieties until they find a way to heal themselves. The right way of healing is not to try to condition their minds with new beliefs, but to inspire them with love of life and to strengthen them to believe only in their inner ability to recover their health. Healing is beyond belief: it is the hope which inspires patients to love themselves to heal themselves, free from emotional neediness or expectation. The following stories illustrates these principles.

One afternoon as I was wandering through Hyde Park I got a call from Scotland. It was my old friend Alice, telephoning me from her home in Edinburgh to ask me for a favour. She wanted me to send absent healing for her husband's slipped disc.

I realised that her husband Peter first of all needed complete rest on a firm mattress for at least ten days while keeping his back immobilised. He had to avoid any movement that might aggravate his slipped disc, and would be cured this way just by following my advice without having to see me.

I was willing to accept Alice's viewpoint that I could cure Peter from a distance by sending him my healing energy, as long as he agreed to immobilise his back. I needed to communicate with Alice in her own language to be able to do my medical work properly, leaving her to believe whatever she wished. The point in the end was to cure her husband, regardless of anyone's beliefs. After his rest in bed had cured Peter it wouldn't matter at all whether it was seen as the result of my absent healing or something else.

"Alice," I replied, "my absent healing for Peter will be effective only when all the conditions are right."

"What do you mean?" Alice sounded puzzled.

"Firstly, Peter needs to stop all his usual activities and do absolutely nothing for ten days. During that time, he must lie with his back straight on a firm mattress on the floor on his right side, with both knees bent at approximately a 45 degree angle. Under no circumstances can he be allowed to move his lumbar area. It should remain straight and immobilised all the time so that I can focus the beam of my healing energy accurately to reach his back and penetrate its tissues perfectly perpendicularly. Only in this way can his back be repaired and healed. Secondly, while Peter is lying completely still on the mattress he must empty his mind of all worry, distraction and anxiety to create space for the full spectrum of my healing energy to fill him with its proper resonance."

"Well, all right…all right," Alice said. She was quiet for a minute.

"Why are you making things so complicated? Can't you please just send us your healing now over the telephone? I know you can; I've often seen you doing it and we all know how effective it is. Please just do it now!"

"Alice," I replied, "Peter has to do what I told you or there is no point in trying to help him. My absent healing can't work and will be useless unless he does exactly as I said. Prepare him to follow the process to receive instant healing. Just do as I say and then I can come and visit you. You know I love and miss you both; Peter has to do what I said. Let me repeat: Peter must do what I told you or there'll be no absent healing and he'll need surgery. Make sure he follows my instructions to the letter and I promise I'll visit you soon."

"Yes, of course, my dear. We're so much looking forward to seeing you. I'll put Peter straight to bed and will make sure he doesn't move a muscle till you arrive."

She did as she was told. A month later Alice called me again, thrilled with the results. Her husband was completely cured and she warmly invited me to Edinburgh for the weekend. Looking forward to seeing my old friends again to share their good news, I booked a first-class return ticket from London to Edinburgh and arrived at Alice and Peter's Georgian house at midday.

As I entered the hall I saw several people looking at me with strange respect. Alice welcomed me excitedly, exclaiming, "Before you meet everyone for lunch I want to show you something extraordinary." She grabbed my hand and took me into a bedroom.

"Look, do you see that mattress on the floor? That's our Mattress of Happiness!"

"What on earth are you talking about?" I asked her in astonishment.

"OK," she laughed, "I'll tell you!"

"This mattress performs miracles. My husband stayed on it for ten days just as you told him to, and it completely cured him." I smiled as she carried on.

"When I told my relatives how it had healed Peter they got so excited that they all wanted to try it out for themselves. They were the people you met in the hall. The tall white-haired man is my uncle; he used it and was cured of asthma. The lovely woman in blue is my sister-in-law Anne, who was cured of endometriosis with acute period pain.

"The short young bald fellow is my nephew Tommy. His gastritis disappeared after only three hours on it. The sweet-

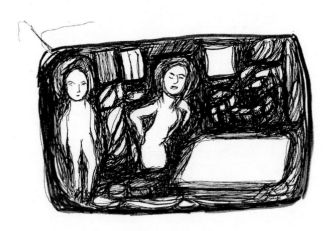

looking young girl is my niece Jasmine. She was healed of migraine and back pain after spending a night on it. She woke up in the morning from a wonderful dream, filled with a new beauty and vitality."

"Incredible! Marvellous! Wonderful!" I exclaimed. "Can I sleep on it tonight? I've got a headache."

"Of course you can!" laughed Alice. "It's your mattress filled with your energy, which healed my husband and whole family."

"What does my energy have to do with this mattress?" I said wearily.

Alice giggled. "Remember last time you were here three years ago? When you spent the weekend with us, you slept on this same mattress and left it filled with your healing energy. When you told me how Peter needed to prepare himself to receive your absent healing and had to sleep on a mattress on the floor, I put him straight onto it and your magic energy in it healed him."

A week after my return home, Georgina, a thirty-three old Londoner, telephoned to ask me to solve her medical problem. When I asked her how she knew about me, she told me that she had heard gossip at her Mayfair hair salon that I was a famous healer who works with angels. She started to describe how attractive, rich and sick she was, with swollen, painful breasts and no periods for three months. She thought that either she was pregnant or a spirit had stopped her periods.

I listened carefully to what Georgina had to say and then gave her my intuitive telephone diagnosis. She was simply feeling the symptoms of a false pregnancy due to temporary prolactinaemia. Stress had caused her uterus to contract, which her brain had wrongly interpreted as a pregnancy. Her pituitary gland responded by secreting large amounts of prolactin and her breasts might have become slightly swollen.

I calmed her down and said all she needed was a blood test. In three months her symptoms would disappear and her body return to normal. If doctors tried to persuade her she had a pituitary tumour she should ignore them.

She didn't take me seriously and decided instead to visit her friend Doris, a medium who channelled the spirit of an ancient Chinese doctor called Chan.

Chan confirmed my intuitive diagnosis. He agreed that she was fine and had no serious health problem. Because she so badly wanted to have a baby, her body had responded by displaying all the symptoms of pregnancy.

She didn't take Dr Chan seriously, either, and after doing the rounds of every available psychic and alternative therapist in her health quest she finally decided to visit her local general practitioner. After listening kindly for over half an hour to her endless complaints, he sent her for tests.

They showed very high levels of prolactin with no signs of pregnancy. As soon as her GP saw the test results he diagnosed her with prolactinaemia caused by a tumour of the pituitary gland. With no further comments or questions and looking weary, he abruptly referred her to an oncologist as a matter of the utmost urgency.

Suddenly all her fears erupted with their attendant phantoms of illness. She was overcome with panic and went straight to hospital like a lamb to the slaughter to ask for brain surgery and radiation before it was too late. At the reception she was referred to Dr George W, a famous young oncologist originally from Beirut. Full of charm, he welcomed her with his perfect smile and she loved his energy. Noticing how elegantly he was dressed, she felt great trust in him. As she told him her story his smile disappeared and the shadow of a frown crossed his handsome face. He gently placed his hand on her shoulder, smiled sympathetically and calmly spoke.

"Georgina, your case is very serious. You need to be admitted to hospital immediately to be placed under medical supervision. If a tumour compresses your brain you could die at any time. I'll send you to our emergency ward to keep you under observation and arrange for you to have a blood test, MRI scan and heart tests today. Prepare yourself for possible surgery tomorrow morning at ten.

"I must tell you, however, that there is a slight risk of complications arising from the surgery. You may find later that you have lost your sense of smell, with possible partial paralysis. I think you'll agree that's a risk worth taking to save your life. We'll also organise a course of radiotherapy and chemotherapy for you after surgery to make sure we've completely destroyed your tumour."

Georgina broke out in a cold sweat and became speechless. She finally surrendered, swallowed her pride and meekly prepared herself for surgery the next day.

At eight in the morning Georgina's handsome Doctor George started his day by visiting her for a friendly chat. After he had finished his tea and biscuits, he summoned his assistant to fetch the results of Georgina's tests. As soon as he saw her results he looked startled. As he went on reading his face turned white and he began to stammer.

"There's something wrong here! You gave me someone else's file."

But the assistant was adamant. "I can assure you it's her file. I was with her all the time during the tests and am quite sure I've given you her correct results."

"Then where's the tumour? There are no signs of it on the scan, and the blood test shows only moderately high serum prolactin, much less than the test result she brought with her. Her prolactin level is too low to indicate a tumour." Dr W took a deep breath to empty his mind of any idea of surgery for Georgina.

"Georgina," he said, "the previous blood test from your doctor, for which we are not responsible, showed a very high level of prolactin, clearly indicating the likely presence of a tumour. We had to act accordingly to prepare you for surgery or risk disaster. We cannot afford to take chances with our patients' lives. In your blood test yesterday, the level of prolactin showed that you had no tumour and the MRI scan confirmed it. You are absolutely fine, Georgina. You don't need surgery after all and can go home."

Georgina sprung up wordlessly from her bed with a shriek of laughter, hurriedly pulled on her clothes and rushed from the hospital. She arrived home like a different person, apparently full of joy and free of her obsessions and worries. She shared her good news with family and guests at a celebration party, where she described in great detail the hell she had been through and how she had triumphed over it. She told her story as if she was a war heroine.

And so she was, though her real enemy was herself with all her mental phantoms and nothing else.

One day I was thinking about Georgina and wondered how she was doing. More than three months had passed since we had spoken, so I rang her and left a message on her answer phone. She returned my call within half an hour and started to tell me all about her great adventure.

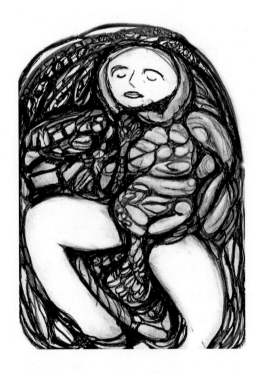

"I felt your presence with me all the time. You were standing by my bed when the surgeon read my test results. I knew you were there to heal me and save me from surgery. I could hear you speaking through the doctor's voice as it became deeper and warmer, saying I was free to go home. You left the room and I rushed to catch you but you had vanished.

"Thank you, thank you, thank you so much! You've always been with me. When you looked at me silently in the hospital I knew you wanted to tell me something but then you were gone and now you know how my heart has been calling for you."

"Georgina, my dear, I have been thinking of you. I'm ready to help you whenever you need me."

"How beautiful! Your words are so full of joy. Where are you calling from? I never imagined anyone like you could exist. We've never actually met and have spoken on the phone only once for a short while, yet I feel so close to you. You really are a great spirit, a true angel. You're behind everything wonderful which has ever happened to me. "

"OK, Georgina," I replied.

"I still have some other medical problems," she said, "can I meet you for a full consultation?"

"No need, Georgina, call me any time, I'm always here."

There was silence and the line went dead.

Healing is inner freedom and true connectedness. We need to be in touch with our inner pain in order to awaken the healer within. Sickness and pain can force us to drop all masks, becoming so free that there is nowhere left to hide.

I need to inspire my patients with healing love, creating therapeutic empathy so as to free them from the misery of their addiction to the outside world – even to me – and to find beauty, freedom and inner peace within themselves. Lady E's story is a good example.

One day a very interesting woman asked me to visit her at home in London. Lady E was forty years old. She suffered from chronic fatigue, insomnia and muscular pain. All her medical tests over the years had been unable to identify any pathology. I examined her and concluded that her suffering resembled a psychosomatic disorder. What was it?

To solve her problem, I needed to develop a good clinical relationship with her. She was extremely attracted to my charisma from our first meeting. We discussed different subjects and I started to understand her better.

She was a very rich woman, brought up like a princess in the highest social circles, an excellent artistic-intellectual personality with tremendous compassion. Her life was full of the beauty of luxury and prosperity. She had everything a human being could want, so why was she suffering?

She was a wonderfully generous spirit and gave a lot of money to help the poor. A member of many charitable organisations, she lectured everywhere in a humanitarian spirit. Full of charm and beauty, she was a brilliant member of the community. Her private life was extraordinary. She was an extremely sensual woman with plenty of handsome admirers. With all this, why was she suffering?

Lady E welcomed me to her magnificent Belgravia apartment with great warmth. I was fascinated by her. She accepted me as I am and guided me with trust into the depths of her soul.

Always eager to serve others, she was addicted to her compassionate daily activities. She had become lost in her idealised self-image and knew how to give better than how to receive. She managed her world well and made it look perfect, but was so busy with outward life that she forgot how to return to herself. As long as she was in the midst of her pleasurable activities during the day she felt uplifted and euphoric. But when she was in bed alone with nothing to do she couldn't calm her anxiety and was prey to insomnia and pain.

Her condition was a type of addiction to tranquillise her anxiety and avoid having to face her inner reality. Lady E had become overshadowed by the outer world. It had absorbed her in pleasurable social life until she lost touch with her inner being and could no longer love herself. I decided to stimulate her spirit and balance her energy to free her from the addictive tendency so she could stand up for the beauty of life within herself. She needed to realise that within her lonely self there lived her healer and lover waiting to overwhelm her with compassion.

Could my healing sessions free her from her addiction to the external world? What would happen when the idols with which she had tranquillised herself fell and there would be nothing left for her to hold on to? I would first have to become her replacement temporary tranquilliser at the moment when her world collapsed and she suddenly found herself facing her emptiness in fear and pain. I would then need to fill her with selfless healing love so that she could confront her painful reality and heal herself by herself.

I had to be fully aware of the possibility that when Lady E dropped her idols her addictive pattern might drive her to idolise me instead as a love guru, making her unable to receive healing. Whatever might happen, I had to allow myself to flow with full trust driven by healing love energy, regardless of all the stages through which her healing process might pass. I had to allow love to do its healing work through me freely. I was certain it would guide her to heal herself independently of me.

I did several healing sessions on the lady. She felt extraordinarily well when I laid my hands on her body. My treatment acted positively on her emotions and provided her with great sensual pleasure. I took this as part of her human feelings! I knelt before her body as if in prayer. Through me was channelled a universal pure love energy that healed her and detached me emotionally. I felt that my patient would gradually find her inner harmony and her emotional nature would become balanced within. But Lady E's healing process was not to occur so readily!

At first she had seen in me a lifesaver, the fulfilment of her artistic, intellectual, romantic and sensual world. Then Lady E started to see me as a messenger sent for her pleasure and inevitably became addicted to me to forget her pain. I understood her and couldn't blame her, but knew that allowing myself to become emotionally involved wouldn't help her.

Lady E felt through me a rich, compassionate universe that was completely new to her. She fell deeply in love with my healing energy and became addicted to it, imagining that it was me she was in love with. I had to open myself to her emotional love in order to transform it with selfless detachment to become her healing consciousness. I had to inspire her to become enlightened along the way, challenging her interior obstacles for her to experience within herself true universal compassion.

I had to help the good lady to find meaning in her life outside her daily affairs.

Lady E started to feel much better and thought I had healed her, but had no confidence in her ability to continue the healing work by herself. She was free of pain and slept well, but was still afraid that her suffering would return if I left her. She wanted me to be with her all the time. For my healing not to become her crutches, she needed to absorb it deeply and make it hers. She had to find her healing lover within herself in order to become emotionally independent.

Was Lady E's addiction to her exterior world really gone? Were her old needy patterns still in her? Was her emotional insecurity still rooted somewhere deep within her, still trying to find a way to tranquillise itself? Perhaps her addiction was still driving her and because she was still unfree she found in me a tastier and more delicious fellow than her routine world could offer.

The time had come to free Lady E from me, to give her breathing space to find herself. I had already strengthened her with plenty of compassionate energy; now she had to learn to use it consciously to continue her healing on her own. The time had come for Lady E to know that she would find her perfect well-being only through my absence and not my presence.

My healing had given her wings but she would not see them. Did she need the wind to hurl her from her nest forcing her wings open to fly freely? I was the healing cocoon in which she grew into a butterfly. How, then, to break myself open for her to fly freely and colour the horizon with her beauty? The wind came when her wings grew and her summer season needed her to sing.

It blew upon me, blowing me far away from her to my country, Lebanon.

I had to leave because my temporary UK visa had expired. To stay longer I had to apply for residency and invest at least two hundred thousand pounds sterling in the country. I didn't have the money and had no other choice but to leave for Lebanon. Only after another two years was I allowed to apply for a new tourist visa. I did my best to convince her that she was cured. No need of me any more! I had to leave the country.

She was deeply shocked.

"God has sent you to me," she said tearfully, "I need you here all the time by my side to support me. I owe you my life. You've brought happiness into it and I don't want to lose you! What will become of me in your absence?"

"You're now in perfect health," I replied. "My clinical examination confirms that you are completely cured and you have demonstrated it by telling me that you are no longer in pain. My role is finished. I have done my best for you. Forgive me, but I have to go. There are other patients who need me more than you do." Tears continued to flow down her cheeks and in a choked voice she replied.

"Please don't leave me! I still have pain at night in my bed, feeling so lonely without you beside me passing your warm hands over my body. As soon as I see you or hear your voice I feel well, but if you leave me alone I know I'll fall ill again."

"My dear lady, my treatment has given you all the energy you'll ever need and plenty of strength to overcome all your disorders. I was the remedy for your old problems, but now you're cured I am your new problem. You have become addicted to the remedy. E, wake up and don't put yourself into a position of weakness. You don't need others to give you sympathy or love. You are a strong woman. You have

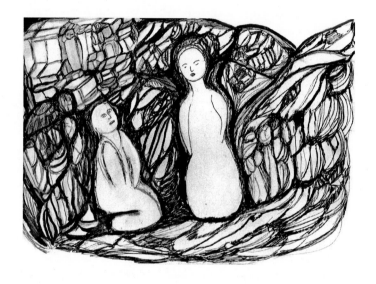

everything. Stand on your own two feet to cast off your feelings of dependence and neediness. Today I am here, tomorrow I no longer will be. You will find instead your healer within. He will heal your pain and give you the pure love you need!"

She stared at me, disturbed and frustrated, rejecting the new reality to which I had exposed her. Sighing deeply, she pleaded with me.

"Why do you have to leave me? How can you do this to me, knowing how much I need and love you? If I'm just another patient to you when you are the only doctor who can help me, why have you made me so completely dependent on you when you know perfectly well that no-one else can replace you? How would other patients like it if you treated them this way? Remember also, dear doctor, that your medical skills are urgently required by my many influential friends to whom I have recommended you. You need to establish fully your unique healing skills within our community. I have now made the decision to sponsor your work and to build upon it a great foundation through which all humanity will be served."

"The decision is not mine," I replied firmly. "I have to leave this country; many poor people elsewhere are in urgent need of my healing medical practice."

"Please don't be so stupid," she sighed, "you absolutely must stay here. This is where you belong. All of us love you. We can't allow you to leave. Our life depends completely on you!" She was silent for a few seconds and then her face brightened. "Wait here a moment." She disappeared, leaving me on my own with a cup of tea.

I wondered why I had told her about my decision to leave England. It had nothing to do with her. How could I help her to realise that she no longer needed me and had to free herself by any means from all dependency?

Lady E came back into the room. She was beaming and walking on tiptoes with a spring in her step. She took my right hand to her bosom, opened it gently and placed a pink envelope into it.

"This is for you to support your patients and your healing message. Take it! This is my present to you for healing me. It's for your foundation to bring your healing love to the world."

I opened the envelope. It contained a cheque for two hundred thousand pounds made out in my name, the exact amount the Home Office needed to allow me to work and become resident in Britain. My inner voice was telling me strongly, "Fantastic! Take it! Do it! You will be a rich and happy man and be able to sponsor your medical work for the sake of humanity." I was ready to take the money.

But suddenly a storm of anger blew me out of control and I saw myself shaking wildly with the cheque ripped to shreds in my hands.

"Lady E, this is not for me!" I yelled at her. "You're only imagining that I healed you! I've simply enjoyed having a good time with you and I will pay you for it, not you me. I wash my hands of your money! My job here is done and there's nothing else left for me to do with you."

All her adoration of me turned into an explosion of anger. For the first time in her life she was overwhelmed by the intensity of her rage. Nobody before had ever rejected her generosity or so rudely smashed her pride. She started to scream hysterically and kicked me out of her home.

"Get out! Go away! Leave me alone! For God's sake go away! I never want to see you again!"

The forceful rejection of Lady E's money had triggered within her a tremendous energetic healing shock which completely smashed all her defence mechanisms, opening her up at last to reconnect herself to her own higher healing love. I could see it easily, though I hadn't planned for it to happen that way, and I felt a sense of tremendous relief. I left her splendid residence still not fully understanding what had provoked my outburst, feeling a great consolation in my heart as wealth beyond compare rained onto me from above, overwhelming me with bliss.

A few weeks later, before leaving the country, I met Lady E by chance in Kings Road, Chelsea. She ran up to me and touched my arm in silent apology. Looking at me warmly, she spoke.

"I have no words left to say. You changed my life. You opened my heart and swept away my fears and worries. You healed my pain and insomnia. I am so happy and grateful; you have brought me back to God."

Healing Absurdity

Healing can happen gradually or spontaneously. It has no apparent logic or rules and can't yet be fully explained by any theory. When my healing works, it works regardless of whether my medical approach is serious, nonsensical or simply compassionate.

The Story of Eli

Joseph, an old childhood friend, had heard that I possess a special ability to cure the incurable. He was persuaded by others to bring his ten-year-old son Eli to me after having looked everywhere for a cure. Eli had suffered from severe idiopathic thrombocytopaenia from the age of five. This is a bleeding syndrome caused by an accentuated decrease in blood platelets. When all medical possibilities were exhausted he had even been forced to resort to visiting saints' shrines, magicians and wizards.

As soon as Joseph arrived at my clinic with his son, he started to tell me all about the problem. Looking at the boy's body, I saw it was covered with purple spots, the sign of subcutaneous haemorrhaging. I felt that it was beyond my capacity to help such a difficult case, but was reluctant to admit it to avoid disappointing him. I didn't even dare to try to apply my hands to his son's skin in case it exacerbated the bleeding.

I was stuck. I couldn't say yes or no, or even raise my little finger. The only thing I could think of was how to escape.

While Joseph gazed reverently at me, I started shouting and gesturing manically, hoping to scare him off and be left in peace without having to take any responsibility. Given my feeling of helplessness, I thought it more appropriate to let him think I had gone mad rather than make him lose his last shred of hope.

But deep down, I still felt there had to be some way to cure the boy. Should I take the risk, and how?

"Joseph! Joseph! I'm not a saint! I'm not a god! I can't just order God to perform a miracle. Look at me!" I gesticulated wildly, body shaking, lips trembling. "I'm just a crazy, stupid doctor, but you're obviously a wise man who can talk to God and tell Him what He should do."

Joseph tried to stay calm at my outburst and smiled. "Put your hands on my son and bless him with your healing."

"What are you talking about? Ask someone else to put his hands on him, not me. I can't do it - as soon as I touch him his bleeding could increase. I'm not allowed to; if I do, something unexpected might happen to make things worse. Stop talking, Joseph, things don't work like this. You've talked enough; you're not the patient and should keep quiet. Shut up! I don't want you or anyone else telling me what to do. I don't need such stupidity. Your son is the patient, not you. It's for him to tell me about his problem."

Joseph was shocked by my attitude and thought I had gone completely mad. He had never expected an old friend like me to behave so rudely and found it hard to understand what lay behind my frustration. Irritated by my failure to meet his expectations, he looked at his son and winked as if to tell him to have no more to do with me. Turning his back on me, he walked towards the door leaving me with Eli and, turning on his heel, he glared at me and said angrily, "Here's your son, do what you like with him."

I looked at Eli and asked him, "Are you really my son?" The boy started to cry.

"I just want to be well. I've had enough of my father's worrying. He's so obsessed with my health. I'm fed up with him dragging me from one hospital to another and from one shrine to another. He never lets me play with other children because he's afraid I might fall over and bleed to death. Doctor, please help me!"

"My hands might not help you. They could make things worse."

"I don't care, try anyway. Whatever happens will be for the best. Just being here with you already makes me feel better." I could hear a new confidence in his voice. He started to talk calmly and firmly to his father, who was still standing in the doorway.

"Father, you don't have to worry about me any more. Just leave me here with the doctor and everything will be fine."

I started to feel very worried. My escape strategy had failed completely. I had been outwitted by a ten-year-old schoolboy and quickly had to come up with another trick before it was too late. All I could think of was to apply the lightest possible touch to his skin, a harmless ineffectual strategy which would satisfy his emotional need.

"OK," I said, "we can try two sessions, today and tomorrow. Then get a new blood test to see whether there's any improvement. If so, we can continue the sessions; if not there'll be no point in coming back." I felt relieved to have come up with a medically convincing diplomatic ploy to avoid having to take any responsibility. I was a hundred percent certain that there would be no change in his condition, but still had to endure two bogus sessions before I could escape Joseph and Eli's wishful fantasies.

As soon as I started to touch the purple spots of subcutaneous bleeding on Eli's body I was surprised to see them beginning to vanish. My first thought was that this was a normal response to light massage and was only temporary.

Three days later Joseph returned to my clinic. Had he brought me his son's blood test to tell me that there was no sign of improvement in his case? Perhaps he wanted to show me that my treatment had failed and would continue to frustrate me with his endless demands. I rushed into the reception room, ready to kick him out of my clinic. I don't need a laboratory test to prove that I'm stupid.

"Joseph, what are you doing here? I did my best for your son and can do no more. Please get out of my clinic and leave me in peace." He smiled and said: "OK, here's the blood test; I'll leave you to read it and then I'll be back."

"I'll read it when you're gone, but you don't need to come back. My secretary will call you to give you the results."

Joseph left at last. I looked at the test results and was astonished to see an extraordinary improvement in Eli's blood platelet count. It had previously been 10,000 and was now 160,000, almost normal. Overcome with excitement, I hurried to the telephone and called Joseph to tell him to come to the clinic immediately. As he entered the door I apologised for my rude behaviour and told him the wonderful news about Eli's cure. We embraced each other and both of us burst into tears of joy.

Twenty years have passed since Eli was cured and he is still doing fine.

The Story of Adi

A twelve-year-old Romani boy called Adi had been suffering from nephrotic syndrome with proteinuria and oedema. His case was an early stage of renal insufficiency.

Adi's parents had heard gossip that I performed miracles. As soon as they received the news, and without stopping to ask whether it was true or not, they picked up their son and rushed with him to see me. As soon as I clapped eyes on them I knew from the expression on their faces that they were emotional fanatics, obsessed with finding a way to catch me so that I would come up with a miracle for their son. How to confront such a situation?

Once again, I was really trapped. Adi's problem was completely beyond my medical competence. I didn't believe I had any healing abilities in this instance, and even if I had I knew they weren't going to work. I felt if I tried to speak honestly about Adi's illness his parents would refuse to listen. All they wanted from me was a miracle.

I was convinced there would be conflict if I told them that I couldn't cure Adi, so any kind of objective dialogue was out of the question. But even though I couldn't talk truthfully to them, I still had to be true to myself.

How could I possibly work on Adi, knowing that nothing could be done for him? It was nonsensical for me to try to find a way to cure him. Having avoided entering into conflict, either with these clients or with myself, I decided to apply my nonsense medicine on Adi, believing deeply that I would be doing absolutely nothing for him and willing to accept whatever might happen, because it was clear to me that it was all nonsense anyway.

As I listened to Adi's parents complaining about their frustrations and flattering me as if God had sent me especially for them, I started to feel that I was a nothing, willing to accept their nonsense and to treat all of them with my own nonsense. They sounded as if they were talking about someone else they were dreaming about, not me, and my only possible response was to be a nothing within myself. All I could do was smile, put my hands on Adi and laugh, whether it was healing or not.

Turning towards him, I chuckled and tapped him on the shoulder cheerfully, feeling just like a useless, happy nonsense doctor.

"Adi, I am the God-sent doctor here to help you and to order Him to produce a miracle especially for you today! As soon as you came through the door with your mother and father, God spoke to me about you in great detail and ordered me to help you. He told me that He sent you here and has given me His great power to perform a healing miracle for you. I thank God for sending you to me. I am so lucky to have you here. You are my honoured guest! Soon you'll be rewarded with the most extraordinary healing and happiness. Amen!"

His parents fell silent and stretched out their hands towards me, crying out, "Bless us with your healing miracles, Doctor, and God will repay you fully for everything you are going to do for us!" I addressed Adi again.

"My son, accompany me now to my holy room. Soon the Healing Spirit from Above will descend upon you to fill you with great Healing Power. You will be a hero! I am so proud of you. You are so special! Chosen by God! A hero! Adi, Adi, Adi! Now you're being cured and soon the whole world will know of it and will be proud of you."

I went with Adi to my room, which had nothing in it except my unmade bed, a pile of dirty clothes and two paintings of naked women on the wall.

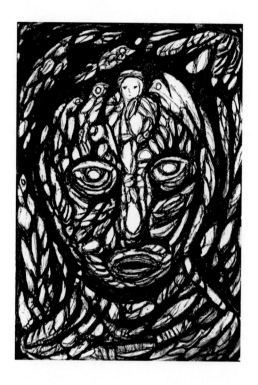

I was surprised to see how easily I had become a great master of lies. How could I act with such self-importance and grandiloquence when I am in myself a nothing who has nothing to do with miracles, a nonsense? How well I play the emotional crook! Am I really such a quack, a senior graduate of the college of higher charlatanism? But I had to play the role of trickster to heal Adi - it well befits me.

It didn't matter whether what I told Adi and his parents were lies or not. They liked it. It was what they wanted to hear. It would change nothing. My inner nonsense doctor would remain a zero. Regardless of any fancies I could cook up and whatever charming lies I might invent, for sure my pigs would never fly.

I laughed at myself. Nothing in me should be taken seriously. My inflated lies to Adi and his parents made me sound delirious. Who cares? However I behave, there is no up or down because I am within myself a zero and live in the reality of my nothingness with great pleasure.

I awoke and called out to myself, "All right, my boy, go and play with Adi, he is such a lovely young chap! I wish I had a son just like him." I put Adi to bed, patted him on the head and left him to sleep.

Twenty minutes later I returned to wake him up and tell him that I had filled him with healing energy and he would be cured. He left me to rejoin his parents, who were waiting in my living room. They had eaten all my fruit and drunk two bottles of my best wine. They felt they were obliged to, since they believed that whatever they could steal from me was blessed.

Two months later, Adi's parents announced that their son had completely recovered from his kidney problem so there was no need for him to see me again.

What joy at last to be free of them. God bless them and keep them away!

My Nephew's Story

While I was still in London my sister-in-law Antoinette telephoned me, crying with the bad news that something really tragic had happened to her nineteen-year-old son Elias.

My nephew Elias was playing volleyball for his sports club one day. He fell onto his left forearm and broke it, fracturing his ulnar. The orthopaedic doctor recommended surgery to fix the fracture with a metal pin. While in hospital, Elias caught an infection during the surgery which spread to the bone. His surgeon prescribed a three-month course of antibiotics to cure the infection, but it didn't work. The only thing left was to perform another operation to clean out the infection and remove the pin.

During the second operation, doctors discovered that one inch of infected bone around the pin had become necrotic. They removed the damaged tissue and cleaned and sterilised the area. Hoping for new bone growth to fill the one-inch gap and knit the fracture, the surgeon then clamped the two broken ulnar sections together with an external metal fixator.

Three months later there was no improvement in Elias' arm – in fact it was getting worse. The infection was still there and had spread to his bone marrow. The surgeons thought a bone graft might be the solution, but it wouldn't have worked because the infection remained, the necrosis had increased and no medical intervention could cure it. If a bone graft had been attempted in Elias' case it would certainly have led to serious complications.

With or without a bone graft, it was inevitable that Elias' hand would have to be amputated. I had to intervene quickly; only a miracle would save his arm now. I was confident that God would not refuse me, knowing how much I love my nephew. He would intervene and help me to save his life.

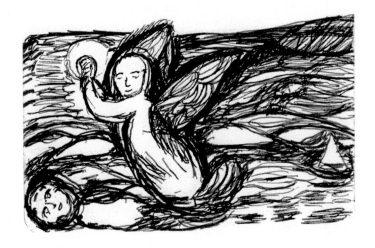

I rushed to Heathrow Airport to catch the next flight to Beirut. As soon as I arrived at our family home and saw Elias we all burst into tears. I was up all night thinking about him, unable to sleep a wink. I felt so helpless, sad and impatient to help. I badly wanted inspiration from anywhere.

And then it came.

In the middle of the night I got up and went straight to Elias to rouse him from sleep. He looked at me surprised and slightly irritated and asked me what was happening; why had I woken him up? "Give me your hand," I told him, "I've come for it! Something woke me up compelling me to see you immediately. Give me your forearm. I have to look for something there."

He smiled and said, "Uncle, do whatever you feel like. You're as crazy as ever!" I grabbed his hand, vibrated it gently for a few minutes and let it go with a laugh. "Elias," I said, "your problem is so simple for me. I can fix it easily." He starred at me suspiciously, convinced that I was completely deluded.

That morning Elias woke up in a state of euphoria, without any anxiety or fear. Looking in the mirror to see what was going on, he felt as beatific as if angels had suddenly abducted him out of space and time. My image suddenly popped into his mind and he called me, full of excitement.

"Uncle, strange things are happening to me. Last night, after you left, I went to sleep feeling as frustrated as if it was the end of the world, but I've now just woken up feeling blissful. Am I going mad? I can't stop smiling. Is it normal for someone facing amputation to feel like this? Tell me, Uncle! Am I normal?"

"It is more than normal," I replied, "it is super-normal. Something extraordinary is happening and I'm coming to you right away to heal your hand!"

I was incredibly excited and felt that the time had arrived at last for my nephew's healing. It looked as if his consciousness had shifted and I could heal him right now!

He welcomed me with tears of joy. My niece Carol was there with her husband Karl, who had come to see what on earth I could possibly do to repair Elias' bone. I hugged him and we started to talk, both of us filled with love.

"Can you raise your hand above your head?" I asked him. He tried, but his forearm started to tremble so uncontrollably that he couldn't lift it more than a few inches. "Ha-ha!" I chuckled, "now you're going to see with your own eyes the miracle your old uncle is about to do for you. Within twenty minutes I'll have you lifting heavy weights with that arm as much as you like – in fact, you'll see that it has become even stronger than the other one!"

Carol, listening to what I was saying to her brother, thought that I'd lost all sense of reality and was talking utter nonsense. She looked at Karl and wagged her finger at her head, saying pityingly, "Poor Uncle Rached has finally gone completely mad! I'm really shocked and frustrated... not only does my brother's hand have to be amputated but uncle's brains are fried...we are such an unlucky family, I simply can't stand it! Let's get out of here."

She burst into tears, shook her head again and rushed out with her husband, leaving me alone in the room with Elias.

I held him close to me, touched his damaged left forearm and got to work on it; it was incredibly weak, almost incapable of any movement. Its muscles had atrophied and it showed extensive pitting from the infection, all the way to the bone. Within fifteen minutes his hand had stopped trembling, the pits on his forearm were filled and the muscles recovered. All signs of his injury had vanished.

It was the most wonderful healing session I've ever had in my life. We were both so drunk with happiness that neither of us could stop laughing joyfully as we watched the miracle of the forearm being cured. I humorously ordered him to pick up and carry a huge heavy bottle of methane gas weighing about twenty kilograms. He took a deep breath, got up, went over to it and grasped it with his newly-healed hand, looking at me questioningly. "Go on, go on, pick it up!" I told him. "Lift it as high as you can! I know you will."

Just as he was starting to raise it his mother, Antoinette, entered the room together with Carol. When they saw Elias lifting the heavy bottle they cried out in fear, "Elias, Elias, please don't listen to your uncle, he's gone quite crazy. Put that bottle down at once!"

But instead of putting down the bottle, Elias started to laugh and lifted it all the way up to his shoulder. Settling it down, he jumped towards me, grabbed my left hand and began arm-wrestling with me. I was amazed at how easily he beat me, and how my prophecy that his left arm would become stronger than the right one had so soon been realised.

Seeing how confused Carol and Antoinette were becoming with all this, I went over to comfort them. We embraced each other joyfully, speechless and tearful. By now, it was evident to all of us that Elias' arm had been cured and the one-inch ulnar gap completely filled. He started to jump up and down. "Uncle," he exclaimed, "it's astonishing! How could I have just lifted that bottle and arm-wrestled with you?"

"Because your bone is mended."

"How did you do it?" he asked.

"Well, I materialised a new bone for you and inserted it into the space of the fracture. Now all you need to do is go to hospital tomorrow for an X-ray to confirm that the bone is fully fused. Show it to your orthopaedic surgeon; when he sees that your bone is healed I'm sure he'll allow you to go and play volleyball and lift weights. I cured your arm and made it better than ever, even stronger than your right arm. You now have an iron arm!"

Next morning the hospital radiologist took a new set of X-rays of Elias' arm and sent them to the surgeon. Several days later the surgeon telephoned Antoinette in a state of total confusion. He told her he wanted Elias back in the hospital to do some more X-rays because he'd seen something strange in the last ones.

Once again, the new X-rays showed that the bone was completely healed. The surgeon called my nephew to ask him how his arm had been cured. When Elias told him his story, the surgeon furtively told him to go home and not to return.

The radiographic image showed that the one-inch gap separating the two halves of Elias' broken ulna had been perfectly filled with new bone tissue. Doctors had never seen anything like it in their lives and had no idea how the new tissue, which the X-ray showed had the density of ivory, could have grown.

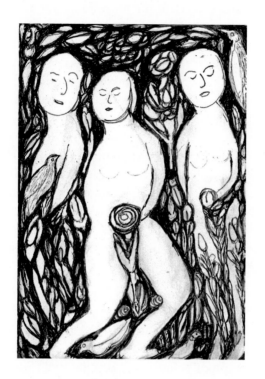

Finally

The ability to heal ourselves is inborn within all of us, whether we are aware of it or not. It is our inner guide that heals us, and all we are required to do is to be open to it and not to allow anything to interfere with it, particularly our own negative emotions and thoughts.

It is not entirely clear how this self-healing takes place, but it is through a homeostatic mechanism that we reconnect with the natural order of the universe within us. It is not easy to reach real healing on one's own. One has to pass through several stages of consciousness. Throughout the process, any obstacle which could obstruct communication and connectedness, whether physical, emotional, mental, psychosocial or spiritual, has to be dissolved. We usually need an external stimulus in the form of another human being or an event. Such inspiration often comes from another person who has already passed through all these stages, whose enlightenment and charisma can trigger within others the processes required to awaken their healing consciousness. One has to find the right healing chemistry, the right therapeutic relationship, so that the hormones of empathy and other neurotransmitters can stimulate healing.

When healing consciousness is activated, a neural web forms which encodes a healing program. Genes can then be turned on or off for the organism to restore itself to health. The development of healing consciousness is a complex process involving psychosocial interactions and bio-transformations within mind and body. Our disconnectedness and disharmony (homeostatic disequilibrium or disease) are healed only when we connect naturally with the original life energy, the roots of universal compassion, for the sake of universal harmony (wellbeing). We need to open up consciousness, to live in our true being in order to heal all disconnectedness and disharmony.

A dramatic shift of consciousness can be seen in patients when they are healed apparently miraculously. This may involve the growth of new bone and tissue, almost instant disappearance of tumours, the cure of paralysis, blindness, deafness and so on. At such moments, patients naturally and spontaneously enter an ecstatic healing trance beyond the physical. They become one with their inner universe, fall in love with themselves and their consciousness expands beyond space and time. Such shifts in consciousness challenge the laws of nature and entropy reverses; it is then not unusual for human body tissue to materialise or dematerialise.

Patients' healing consciousness has to be awakened. Everyone has his or her unique methods, beliefs and language needed for such a process. It varies from one individual to another, depending on their culture, education, personal capacities and so on. Healing can be seen as a kind of revelation or inspiration, transforming conscious and unconscious negative emotions and memories into positive, creative and harmonious ones. It may be experienced as a mystical insight or spiritual process, by which the mind-body is enabled to achieve a state of harmony and well-being.

Healing is a living language within us, a voice crying through matter. It is the everlasting symphony of life playing its music deep within us. We listen to its beauty and melt into the consciousness of the universe.

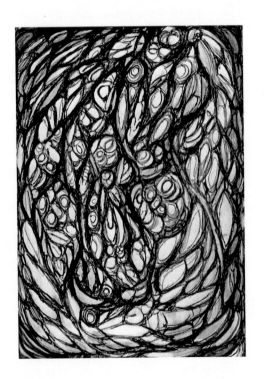